THE COMPLETE HANDBOOK OF

HEALTH TIPS

BASED ON THE LATEST NUTRITIONAL AND SCIENTIFIC FINDINGS AND TIME-PROVEN REMEDIES

BY
R. EMIL NEUMAN

Published By
United Research Publishers

THE COMPLETE HANDBOOK OF
HEALTH TIPS
BASED ON THE LATEST NUTRITIONAL AND SCIENTIFIC FINDINGS AND TIME-PROVEN REMEDIES

ISBN 0-9614924-1-4

Printed in U.S.A.

Order additonal copies of The Complete
Handbook of Health Tips from:

United Research Publishers
P. O. Box 2344
Leucadia, CA 92024

Full 30-day money back guarantee if not satisfied.

Introduction

This book contains a treasury of health information drawn from the latest medical and nutritional literature and time-proven remedies.

The book is arranged by subject matter. Each topic is covered in a clear, concise manner. You can quickly scan through the book and focus in on topics of particular interest to you. However, I urge you to read the entire book. It gives a wealth of interesting and valuable health information of vital importance to you and your family.

In addition to hundreds of health tips the book gives you toll-free telephone numbers you can call to get Free, up-to-date information on most any health subject. A trained specialist will be available to answer your questions or send you helpful information. The book also contains telephone numbers to get specific information on matters such as getting a second opinion on surgery, cancer, impotence and many other subjects.

While the book should prove to be an extremely valuable source of health information, an important caution should be fully understood: This book is not intended to be a substitute for medical advice from a doctor. Don't attempt to self-diagnose a medical condition or embark on self-treatment of a serious ailment. This can be dangerous. Seek the best medical treatment when needed.

The book contains a section that will help you find the most competent medical advice available in your area. It will tell you where and how to find the right doctor for your individual medical needs.

Please enjoy the book and I wish you the very best.

CONTENTS

SECTION I

HEALTH
TIPS

ACNE

Avoid Acne Flareups Acne is caused by clogging and inflamation of the oil glands and ducts beneath the skin. This causes the acne pimples and blackheads. About 75 percent of adolescent boys and 50 percent of adolescent girls develop acne. The following can cause acne flareups:

• *Cosmetics.* Acne flareups can be due to use of cleansing creams, night moisturizers, face foundations and rouges. These products often contain additives such as fatty acids, coal tars and oils that clog pores.

• *Foods.* Foods and vitamin supplements containing iodine may aggravate acne, says Dr. James Fulton, of the Acne Research Institute, Newport Beach, California.

• *Poor Hygiene.* When dirt and oil build up it can clog pores and cause a flareup.

Home Care Suggestions

• For mild to moderate cases of acne, benzoyl peroxide is recommended. Benzoyl peroxide is available at most drug stores. It unclogs skin pores and stimulates new cell growth. Rubbing ice cubes on the face for 3 minutes before applying medication helps, according to Dr. James Fulton of the Acne Research Center in California. Ice reduces inflamation. Wrap ice in a wash cloth to avoid freezing hand.

• The traditional treatment for acne had been the antibiotic tetracycline. However, a Swedish study showed zinc to be as effective as tetracycline and does not have the side effects. A study performed in Sweden gave 19 acne patients 135 milligrams of zinc a day and a second group of 18, 750 milligrams a day of tetracycline. After 12 weeks both groups showed a 67% improvement in their complexion. It is believed that zinc works to clear acne by reducing irritation and inflamation and by helping the damaged skin heal itself. Consult your physician before taking zinc supplements.

• Research has shown that a low zinc diet can bring on acne flareups in 10 to 14 days. Be sure your diet provides adequate

amounts of zinc. Foods rich in zinc include sea food, spinach, mushrooms, whole grains and sun flower seeds.
- Many persons have reported that applying vitamin A from capsules helps acne flareups.

Acne Hotline For information on causes and cures of an acne condition, there is a toll-free number you can call. Call 1-800-235-ACNE (1-800-225-ACNE in California). A trained specialist will be available to answer your questions on acne.

AIR TRAVEL

Reducing Pressure In Ears Many people experience extreme discomfort while flying in an airplane. This pain is caused by air pressure in the cabin creating a vacuum in the middle ear. The pain can get very severe unless something is done to balance the air pressure in the middle ear.

What To Do To Avoid Discomfort
- Many people get relief by chewing gum or sucking on mints. Swallowing air while chewing the gum tends to balance the pressure in the middle ear.
- When chewing gum does not work many people get relief by closing their mouth and pinching the nose shut and gently blowing out their cheeks. If a clicking noise is heard this means the procedure was successful.
- If these measures do not result in relief right away keep on trying them.

ALCOHOLISM (See also HANGOVERS)

Tips For Minimizing Alcohol Effects Heavy alcohol use can cause hepatitis, cirrhosis of the liver, gastritis (a painful inflamation of the stomach lining), neuritis

2

(inflamation of the nerves) and vitamin deficiencies.

Heavy drinking may be worse than cigarettes in contributing to oral cancer. Researchers say that people who smoke 40 cigarettes a day stand a five times greater risk of getting oral cancer than non-smokers. But people who drink 6 ounces of whiskey a day run a 15.2 times greater risk of getting oral cancer than non-smokers, according to Dr. Arthur Mashburg and Dr. Lawrence Garfinkel. Here are some suggestions for minimizing the harmful effects of alcohol:

• Drinking alcohol depletes the body of vitamins, especially vitamin B, says Dr. Boras Tabakoff, Director of the Alcoholism and Drug Abuse Research and Training Program at the University of Illinois Medical Center. When drinking, take a vitamin B-complex.

• To help prevent a hangover from alcohol consumption take one 50 milligram B-complex tablet before going out. Also take one while you're drinking. This will help replace the B vitamins that alcohol destroys in your body.

• Excessive alcohol can spark a zinc deficiency by flushing stored zinc out of the liver. Insufficient zinc can cause prostate troubles and problems with sex, says Dr. Carl Pfeiffer, from the Bio-Brain Center, Princeton, New Jersey. Supplement your diet with zinc when drinking heavily.

• Other nutrients destroyed by alcohol are magnesium, vitamin A, C, D, and calcium. Just two or three drinks per day will start to deplete these nutrients. It's a good idea to take a multi-vitamin daily when drinking heavily.

ALLERGIES

How To Live With An Allergy An allergy is a reaction or sensitivity to a substance in the environment called an allergen. Common symptoms of allergy are watery eyes, runny nose, itching and inflamed skin. Other symptoms include headache, sinus stuffiness and a host of other ailments. As many as 1 in 5 Americans suffer some kind of allergy.

We get allergic reactions from breathing air containing allergens, touching things with allergens and eating foods having allergens.

Identifying the specific allergens that cause reactions may be time consuming, painful and expensive. Often, specific allergens are never discovered.

Avoiding Allergens In The Air Allergies can be avoided by minimizing exposure to common allergens in the air. Here are some tips from the American Academy of Allergies, Public Education Committee:

- Avoid ragweed, sage brush, pig weed, tumble weed, Russian thistle and cockle weed in the fall.
- On windy days during the pollen season do not play golf, hike, horseback ride or jog.
- Minimize early morning outdoor activity. Pollen generally is emitted from sunrise to 10 a.m. If you drive to work during those hours keep your windows closed.
- Don't install a window fan. It will exhaust house air and bring in allergens through open windows. Instead, install a central or window air conditioner which will recirculate air in the rooms where windows are shut.
- Dust daily with chemically treated or oil dust cloth so you won't just spread the dust around.
- Vacuum carpets and rugs daily changing the vacuum bags frequently.
- Keep pets away from the general living area. Never let them sleep in the bedroom, especially on your bed.
- A cat's litter box is a prime source of allergens.
- Enclose your pillow, box spring and mattress in plastic. This will reduce dust and mites that can trigger an allergic reaction.
- Keep your bedroom free of objects that collect dust. This

would include magazines, books, stuffed animals and knick knacks. Dust and vacuum frequently.

• Keep house plants out of your home. They can trigger an allergic reaction from molds that form on them when they are wet.

• Try using an artificial Christmas tree. Live trees contain hydrocarbons that can carry molds and be irritating.

• Keep your grass trimmed short. No taller than 1 inch. This reduces exposure to grass pollen.

• Do not use aerosol sprays.

• If your home has a forced-air heating system try putting a cheese cloth over the vent. This will act as a filter and catch most of the dust.

• If possible get an air-conditioner unit for your home.

Testing For Allergens In Things To determine whether you may be allergic to some kind of fabric or material place a small piece of fabric or material in a jar and place the jar in the sun or warm place for several hours. Then remove the lid and smell the air in the jar. Keep track of any reactions you may experience. If you have no symptoms, you are probably not allergic to that item in the jar.

Identifying Food Allergies Millions of people are allergic to certain foods and don't know it. But there is a simple test you can do to identify allergen foods, says Dr. Arthur F. Coca, allergist and immunologist. Dr. Coca recommends taking your pulse before and after meals. For example, let's say you suspect that you may be allergic to oranges. One morning, take your pulse when you get up. Then eat an orange. Wait 30 to 60 minutes, then take your pulse again. See if there's any abnormal increase in your pulse rate. While this test is not 100% accurate, in a large number of cases an increase in pulse rate indicates an allergy to a food or substance. To take your pulse, lightly press two or three fingers on your wrist. Do not use your thumb because your thumb has a pulse of its own.

Foods most commonly causing allergies: corn, eggs, fish,

5

milk, nuts, wheat. Foods that often cause allergies: alcohol, berries, buckwheat, cane sugar, chocolate, coconut, coffee, mustard, oranges or citrus fruits, peanut butter, peas, pork, potatoes, soy, tomatoes, yeast.

Look Out For Fruits And Vegetables Pesticides and preservatives on fruits and vegetables can be a prime source of allergens. To remove pesticides, soak the fruit or vegetables in a sink filled with water and a quarter cup of vinegar. Then scrub the fruits and vegetables and rinse them under cold water.

Grain Allergens Grains are a major allergen source. It's a good idea to transfer grain products including rice, flour and cereals into glass or metal containers. This will prevent mold and insect infestation that can cause allergies. Keep the containers in a cool, dry place.

ALZHEIMER'S DISEASE

Research Studies To Consider This is a disorder in elderly persons caused by a degeneration of the blood vessels of the brain, resulting in brain shrinkage. There is a steady decline in brain function, memory and personality. Victims often cannot recognize family members and close friends. Alzheimer's disease affects about 10 percent of persons over age 65. There is no known treatment.

• A preliminary Dutch study evaluated patients with Alzheimer's type senility and alcohol-related brain damage and found low levels of vitamin B-12 and zinc in both groups. Researchers believe that early recognition and adequate treatment with B-12 and zinc can possibly prevent irreversible damage to patients with these disorders. This study was published in the Journal of Orthomolecular Psychiatry.

• In a preliminary research study 10 patients with

6

Alzheimer's disease were given choline in their diets. The average age of the patients was 77. Three of the 10 patients seemed less confused after the choline treatment.

Researchers believe choline may work best before the onset of Alzheimer's disease. When choline was given to patients under 65 with beginning stages of the disease all patients reported improvement in memory. Lecithin is rich in choline. Lecithin is available at most health food stores. This study was reported in the medical journal Lancet.

ANAL ITCHING

How To Avoid Anal Itching Common causes of this condition include intestinal pinworms, hemorrhoids, allergies and eating highly spicy foods. Coffee, tea, colas and chocolate may irritate bowels and cause anal itching, says Dr. Lester Tavel of Pearland, Texas. Most sufferers have excess mucus that seeps through the anal canal keeping the area moist and irritated. Tips to avoid anal itching:

• Keep the anal area dry and clean. Use of oily medications only worsen the condition.

• A dusting powder should be used daily. This is preferable to an antifungal preparation.

• Avoid beverages and foods that contain caffeine.

Yogurt For Itching--A Study To Consider A preliminary study published in "Diseases of the Colon and Rectum" showed people suffering from anal itching were helped by lactobacillus acidophilus. Of the 87 people participating in the study, 74 said that itching completely disappeared or substantially subsided. Researchers recommend adding acidophilus obtained from yogurt to your diet. Both lactobacillus acidophilus or lactobacillus bulgaricus are contained in yogurt. Either will provide the same benefits.

Self-diagnosis can be dangerous. If you have a serious health problem, see your doctor promptly.

7

ANGINA

Cause Of Pain Angina is a pain in the chest caused by a lack of oxygen in the heart. This lack of oxygen is normally caused by a narrowing of the arteries due to cholesterol formation. The pain may feel like indigestion and it may shoot to the arm. Angina occurs whenever the heart requires more oxygen than the narrowed arteries can provide.

Things To Avoid
- Don't engage in sudden, strenuous physical activity. Always warm up first.
- Don't overeat. Eat at regular intervals.
- Rest for 30 minutes after meals, especially heavy meals.
- Sleep in a well-ventilated room.
- Try to avoid constipation.

See your doctor for regular checkups.

Preliminary Research To Consider
- *Vitamin E.* According to Dr. Terence W. Anderson of the University of British Columbia, vitamin E may help angina discomfort. Dr. Anderson conducted a study of 15 angina patients who were already taking vitamin E. Without the patients knowing, 7 were given fake pills containing no vitamin E. After three weeks 3 patients had to drop out of the study because of severe angina pain. A fourth stayed on but complained of increased pain. The remaining 8 who continued taking vitamin E daily had no increase in the angina pain. Foods rich in vitamin E include dark green vegetables, fruits and rice.
- *Aspirin.* Based on a study of 11,965 men having heart conditions, the Federal Food and Drug Administration concluded that it is safe and effective to take one aspirin a day to control angina. Among men suffering unstable angina who took an aspirin each day, the risk of dying from heart attack dropped about one-half.

One regular 325 mg. aspirin should be the daily dose. Of

course, you should continue to see your doctor at regular intervals. Aspirin appears to help prevent clotting of the blood which can cause heart attack. The Food and Drug Administration emphasized that aspirin therapy is not a substitute for other preventative measures such as stopping smoking, eating better, losing weight and sensible exercise.

● *Lecithin/Vitamin E.* Researchers reported treating angina with 800 milligrams and more of vitamin E a day. Favorable responses have been reported with lecithin using 15 grams a day.

● *Amino Acid-L-Carnitine.* Preliminary studies done by Dr. Robert Atkins shows that this amino acid may be valuable in relieving the pain of angina.

● *Tilting Bed.* Many people suffer angina attacks at night. Tilting the head of the bed upward 10 degrees may reduce angina pain. Lying flat increases the amount of blood returning to the heart, reducing oxygen flow. The best way to tilt a bed is to put wooden blocks under front legs.

ANOREXIA NERVOSA

Cruical Anorexia Facts This is an eating disorder that strikes younger women who suppress the urge to eat to the point of malnutrition and even starvation.

● 95 percent of sufferers are female, mostly teens from upper middle class homes.

● It mostly strikes obedient girls who try to overly please parents, teachers and others. This creates a subconscious need to control at least one part of her life--eating.

● Victims often fear growing up so they unconsciously "diet away" physical signs of maturity--curved hips, larger breasts, etc.

● Anorexia sufferers need professional counseling.

Zinc--Preliminary Research One preliminary study

showed that supplements of the mineral zinc were 80% successful in helping sufferers overcome anorexia, says Dr. Douglas Latto, British Nutrition Foundation in London, England. Zinc supplements helped patients regain appetite and put on weight.

When the anorexia victim stops eating the body begins to lose zinc. As the zinc levels in the body go down the sense of taste and smell is destroyed. Without these senses the desire for food declines even further. But when anorexics were given zinc they regained these senses. Their appetites returned and they started eating again. Zinc supplements of more than 50 milligrams per day are not recommended without medical supervision. Foods rich in zinc include sea food, spinach, mushrooms, whole grains and sun flower seeds.

ANTIBIOTICS

Kills Both Bad And Good Bacteria Antibiotics kill the good bacteria in your body as well as the harmful bacteria. Killing off beneficial bacteria can cause diarrhea and other stomach problems. When the beneficial bacteria is destroyed it can cause fungus to grow in the intestines, vagina, lungs and mouth.

When taking antibiotics be sure to take generous amounts of acidophilus culture to help maintain the beneficial bacteria in your body. Acidophilus culture can be obtained through eating yogurt or taking acidophilus capsules. Both are available at most helath food stores and supermarkets.

ANTS

Stopping Ant Attacks Ants may carry germs that can cause disease. To stop ants from crawling into your home through cracks in the walls or sink try putting a little petrolium jelly in the cracks. Also, sprinkle red pepper around the counter tops. Ants can't stand red pepper. Plant mint near your front and back door. Ants do not like mint.

ASPIRIN

Suggestions To Avoid Stomach Upset
● Aspirin will cause less digestive upset if taken after eating food and with a full glass of water.

● Avoid combining aspirin with acidic foods such as citrus fruits and juices, alcoholic drinks. They may increase irritation in the stomach.

● Never take aspirin with vitamin C. This will increase possibility of stomach bleeding.

● Aspirin with an enteric coating reduces irritation to the stomach. The enteric coating delays absorption of aspirin until it reaches the intestine.

ASTHMA

Things That Trigger An Attack This condition is caused by an obstruction of the bronchial tubes brought about by a sensitivity to substances in the environment and other factors. About 3 percent of the U.S. population suffers asthma symptoms.

According to the American Lung Association the most common things that can trigger an asthma attack are:

● Household products such as paint thinner and chlorine bleach.

● Cold and extra humid air.

● Air pollution.

- Exercise.
- Infections caused by colds and viruses.
- Tobacco smoke.
- Emotions such as anger, fear and even happiness.
- Pollen, mold and spores; hair and feathers; and certain foods such as chocolate, nuts and eggs.

Tips On Preventing Attacks

- Avoid food that contains preservatives and dyes such as BHA and BHT, sodium benzoate and the dye known as FD&C yellow #5.
- Avoid aspirin.
- Avoid cola drinks.
- Avoid cold liquids. Cold liquids may shock your bronchial tubes into asthma spasms.
- Keep the air clean in your home. Use air filters to trap dust and mold particles.
- Avoid dogs and cats including short-haired breeds. Dogs and cats give off dander--tiny particles from the hair and skin that can produce reactions.
- Avoid feathered pillows.
- Choose the right kind of carpeting. The backing of many carpets is made of gute, which may induce allergic reactions. Choose foam-rubber backing and padding instead.
- Do not wallpaper bedrooms. Mold can grow behind the paper.
- Buy synthetic Christmas trees. Real trees contain mold.
- Keep windows closed when air pollution is high outside.
- Wear a scarf over your mouth in cold weather, but avoid woolen scarves which may trigger an allergic reaction.

Mushrooms Can Trigger Attack Mushroom spores are released into the open air after mushrooms ripen and have been harvested. If you like mushrooms get the canned ones that are packed in liquid. Most mushrooms release spores once a year in the fall. Cultivated mushrooms release spores the year round.

Stay Away From Salad Bars Many items in a salad bar are treated with bisulfates. These are food preservatives that keep food looking fresh while out in the open for hours at a time. These preservatives can cause serious adverse reactions in persons having asthma. The Food and Drug Administration is aware of about 90 deaths from adverse reactions due to these preservatives.

Getting Relief--Research To Consider

• *Coffee.* A few cups of coffee may relieve asthma symptoms, according to studies conducted at the University of Manitoba in Winnepeg, Canada. Researchers found that the caffeine equivalent to 2 cups of coffee unclogged blocked bronchial passages in the lungs. The study was reported in the New England Journal of Medicine.

• *Vitamin C.* Taking vitamin C may help control asthma attacks. In one study researchers gave asthmatics 1,000 milligrams of vitamin C a day. Those taking vitamin C had about 25% fewer attacks than those who received a fake pill. When the subjects stopped taking vitamin C, they once again suffered the same number of asthma episodes as the people who did not take the vitamin C. This study was published in the Journal of Tropical and Geographical Medicine. Foods rich in vitamin C include citrus fruits and fruit juices, berries, cabbage, green vegetables and potatoes.

• *Vitamin B-6.* In a study of 15 asthmatics given 50 milligrams of vitamin B-6 twice daily, symptoms were relieved in every case, says Dr. Robert Reynolds, a U.S Department of Agriculture research chemist. Foods rich in vitamin B-6 include bananas, cabbage, green leafy vegetables, whole grains and fish.

Deep Breathing Exercise For Relief

Deep Breathing Exercise For Relief According to the American Lung Association, breathing correctly can relieve wheezing, chest tightness and shortness of breath. The following exercise can be practiced lying down, sitting or standing. It should be done daily for maximum benefits.

1. Think of your chest and stomach as a container for air. Breathe in through your nose slowly filling the bottom of the container first. Continue until the stomach feels inflated like a balloon. If you place your hand on the spot just above your naval you can feel your middle rise and fall with each breath. Exhale slowly through your mouth. The container should feel completely empty and your stomach should feel flat before you inhale again.

2. Repeat. Inhale and exhale 12 times.

Relaxing Away An Asthma Attack The American Lung Association teaches children to relax as a way of warding off an asthma attack. The following exercise when practiced for 5 minutes a day can be used whenever the chest starts to feel tight or other signs occur. This exercise works for adults also.

• Stand up and make all your muscles very tight. Then take a deep breath. Point your chin up to the ceiling and grit your teeth. Hold your arms out straight. Keep your elbows tight and your fists tightly closed. Your legs and toes should be stiff. Hold for a few seconds.

• Then let everything go like a balloon that's been deflated. Completely relax all your muscles until you feel like a wet dishrag or noodle.

• Flop to the floor in a lying position and stay there. Close your eyes. Keep your arms limp and loose. Your face and feet should be limp also.

• Picture yourself floating down a river. Concentrate on each muscle and how nice and floppy it feels.

• Breathe softly and easily as if you were fast asleep in your bed. Stay quiet and relaxed and feel how pleasant it is.

• Open your eyes. Turn on the relaxed wet dishcloth feeling whenever you feel nervous or short of breath, or feel an asthma attack coming on.

ATHLETES FOOT

4 Suggestions For Preventing Athletes foot is a fungus infection between the toes and on the balls of the feet. It causes itching, burning and stinging. The skin becomes red and cracks.

Eight out of ten men in America contract athletes foot sometime during their lifetime. Whenever the space between the toes remains moist the fungus can take hold. The fungus can be caught quickly by walking barefoot in a gym or locker room. To avoid problems:

- Wear protective footwear to avoid contact with the floor.
- Dry feet thoroughly with a clean towel--especially between the toes.
- Change socks every day--twice a day in extremely hot weather.
- Use dusting powder to keep feet dry.

Home Care Of Athletes Foot

- Bathe feet several times a day with soap and warm water. Dry feet and sprinkle with Desenex or Tinactin, available at drug stores.
- Several athletes foot preparations are available at drug stores. These include compound undecylenic acid ointment, tolnaftate and miconazole. Directions usually call for morning and night applications until symptoms go away.
- At night separate toes with cotton balls to reduce friction on inflamed skin.
- Wear open toe shoes or no shoes at all in hot weather.

BACK PAIN

17 Simple Tips To Help Prevent Back Trouble
- Don't stand or sit in one position for a long period of time while working.

- While on the telephone avoid holding the telephone between your ear and neck for long periods of time. This can tense the muscles in your shoulder and cause back trouble.

- While driving long distances in your car, stop periodically and take a break. After you've been driving for a while, don't make any sudden movement that could pull a muscle.

- Sleep on a firm mattress. The harder the mattress, the better.

- Use pillows with manufactured fibers. Foam rubber pillows tend to elevate your head higher than it should be, thus crimping your neck.

- Wear comfortable shoes. The higher the heel, the greater the risk of back pain.

- When carrying anything on your shoulder switch the weight to the other shoulder from time to time.

- When lifting, keep your back straight and bend your knees. Let your leg muscles do most of the work. Hold the object you're trying to lift close to your body.

- Never stretch when you're reaching for a high object.

- Don't bend over furniture to open or close windows.

- Always push a large object, never pull it. Pulling places a great strain on the muscles of the lower back.

- While sitting down, keep your knees about an inch higher than your hips. This reduces the strain on your lower and upper back muscles.

- Before doing work spend a few minutes warming up. Warming up exercises should include bending, stretching and twisting.

- When going to bed lie on your side and draw one or both knees up toward your chin. This is a good resting position for your back.

- If you sleep on your stomach, put a pillow under your abdomen so your back is raised slightly. The worst sleeping position for your back is flat on your stomach with your head raised on a pillow.

- When getting out of bed in the morning be careful.

- After sitting or standing in one position for more than 10 minutes, avoid any sudden or forced movement. For example, be careful when you're watching T.V. and the phone rings or when you're driving in your car and you get out suddenly.

BACKYARD BARBEQUES

Safety Tips To Follow An outside barbeque in the backyard can be dangerous, especially with children. The heat intensity from the fire can reach up to 500 degrees. This temperature is the same inside or outside the grill. The following suggestions will help avoid an accident:

- Keep the grill at least 6 feet away from the house.
- Water the ground around the grill lightly before lighting the coals.
- When using lighter fluid, first soak the coals. Then wait 5 or 10 minutes before striking a match.
- Never add more lighter fluid after the fire is blazing.
- Once fire is lit stay in the area to make sure the fire stays under control and children stay away from the grill.
- Wait until the coals are glowing evenly before starting to cook.

BAD BREATH (HALITOSIS)

3 Tips To Avoid Bad breath may be caused by poor mouth hygiene, nose or throat infection, teeth and gum decay, excessive smoking or the presence of bacteria in the mouth. The following suggestions may help avoid bad breath:

- *Acidophilus.* Bad breath is often associated with putrefactive bacteria living on undigested food in the stomach. This condition causes gas to be released through the breath. Supplementing the diet with the friendly bacteria lactobacillus acidophilus often helps. Acidophilus can be obtained from yogurt or in capsule form--available at most health food stores and supermarkets.

• **Brushing Your Tongue.** Dr. Joseph Toncetich from the School of Dentistry, University of British Columbia in Vancouver, Canada, performed a study to find out the best way to reduce bad breath. Eight volunteers, all of whom suffered from morning bad breath, participated in the study. The doctor found that brushing teeth reduced mouth odor about 25%. Brushing the tongue reduced mouth odor 75%. Brushing the teeth and the tongue reduced mouth odor 85%. This study was published in the journal called Oral Surgery.

• **Mouth Washes.** Most contain high concentrations of alcohol. The alcohol kills bacteria in the mouth but only temporarily. When the bacteria returns more come back than before using the mouth wash. Many dentists believe that alcohol-laced mouth wash can damage the tissue in the mouth, cause inflamation and result in bad breath.

BALDNESS

New Drug Offers Hope Researchers at San Antonio, Texas, Health Science Center say a new drug called Minoxidil actually stimulates hair growth on scalps of bald men. Nearly half of 619 people testing Minoxidil experienced moderate to heavy hair growth.

Minoxidil was originally used for controlling high blood pressure. Doctors became interested when patients reported hair growth as a result of using the medicine. Studies are showing the compound is safe with no side effects. Once this drug is approved by the Food and Drug Administration it will cost about $35.00.

BAND-AIDS, REMOVING

Taking The Sting Out Removing band-aids can be very painful, especially on children. The next time you have to remove a band-aid, instead of ripping it off, try using a hair dryer to heat it up. This will soften the adhesive and the band-aid should peel off easily with little or no discomfort.

BED SORES

4 Tips For Avoiding Bed Sores
• Vitamin C. The healing rate of bedsores can be improved by taking up to 500 milligrams of vitamin C a day.
• Use of inflated rubber cushions helps avoid bedsores.
• Shifting body with pillows helps prevent sores.
• Keep bed clothing loose.

BETA-CAROTENE

May Lower Cancer Risk Most of the latest research on cancer focuses on vitamin A in the form of beta-carotene. Research shows low levels of beta-carotene increase risk of lung cancer and other cancers. Beta-carotene is amply found in carrots, dark leafy greens, sweet potatoes, squash and other vegetables. Once inside your body beta-carotene is converted into vitamin A. In getting daily sources of vitamin A, it is better to use beta-carotene supplements than plain vitamin A.

BIO-FLAVONOIDS

Helps Vitamin C Absorption These are compounds found in the white pulp of oranges, grapefruits and other citrus fruits and vegetables. Bio-flavonoids enhance the body's absorption of vitamin C. Studies show that citrus bio-flavonoids seem to favorably alter the way our bodies use vitamin C. It helps concentrate the nutrient in various tissues making it more absorbable, according to the American Journal of Clinical Nutrition.

BIRTH CONTROL PILLS

Users Need More Vitamin B-6 And Folic Acid Research has shown that women taking the birth control pill are often low in the vital nutrient vitamin B-6. The National Research Council reported that 15 to 20 percent of oral contraceptive users show signs of B-6 deficiency.

Birth control pill users also need more folic acid, part of the B-complex vitamins, according to Dr. Daphine Roe, Professor of Nutrition at Cornell University. Foods high in vitamin B-6 include whole grain cereals, wheat germ, vegetables, bananas and meat. Good sources of folic acid include leafy, dark green vegetables, organ meats and citrus fruits.

When taking the pill, be sure your diet provides enough B-6 and folic acid. If you're not sure consider vitamin supplements.

BLISTERS ON FEET

What To Do For Blisters
• Wash the blister thoroughly with soap and water. Let dry.

- Apply a band-aid strip to the blister. Apply other overlapping band-aids until the entire blister and a margin of normal skin is smoothly covered with tape.
- Leave this in place for 5 days then remove. The dead surface of skin of the blister usually hangs limp by this time. You can trim it off with scissors or let it dry.

BLOATING

Suggestions For Relieving Bloating Many women before their menstrual period find themselves puffy and water-logged. Clothes fit too tightly due to temporary gain in water weight. This can be very uncomfortable. The following tips will help avoid bloating:

- Reduce salt intake. Buy a salt substitute or flavor foods with lemon juice, herbs and spices. Avoid salty snack foods like potato chips and pretzels. Carefully check food labels for excess salt content.
- Stay away from foods that cause intestinal gas. Most common offenders are dairy products, nuts and spicy foods like pizza and tacos.
- Avoid cola drinks and chocolate.
- Keep your weight down. Excess fat tissue attracts and stores fluid.
- Avoid emotional stress.
- Avoid alcohol. It makes bloating worse, especially on hot days.
- Wear loose clothing. Avoid belts and tight shoes. Also wear low-heeled shoes. Take off tight rings if your hands swell.
- Avoid water pills. Water pills cause your kidneys to work overtime leading to a loss of important minerals such as potassium, sodium, calcium and magnesium, according to Dr. Milan Pazourek of Tacoma, Washington.

- Drink more water. Drinking 4 to 6 glasses of water a day makes your kidneys work more efficiently.
- Exercising improves vascular tone and circulation.
- Eat natural diuretics like watermelon, strawberries, apples, grapes, beets, asparagus. They stimulate the body to eliminate water.
- Take vitamin B-6. You can take up to 200 milligrams a day during times of pre-menstrual fluid retention. This helps reduce bloating.
- Eat only fish or protein for 2 or 3 meals a day. This will have a diuretic effect on the body.

Anti-Bloat Ingredients Approved By Federal Government's Panel Of Experts Three ingredients were found safe and effective as diuretics by a U.S. government panel of medical experts:

- Ammonium Chloride (Should not be used by anyone with impaired kidney or liver function). Effectiveness diminishes after 4 or 5 days.
- Pamabrom.
- Caffeine.

Drug stores and supermarkets should have products containing these ingredients. Use diuretics only when all other measures fail to bring relief.

BLOOD PRESSURE

What Is Blood Pressure Blood pressure is the force of the blood against artery walls which carry blood throughout the body. Blood pressure is measured using two numbers. The first number is your systolic pressure. This is the larger number. It measures the force of your blood against artery walls when the heart has contracted and is gushing blood throughout the body. Think of the systolic pressure as a garden hose measuring the force in your arteries when the water is turned on. The second number measures the diastolic pressure. This is the force of the blood against the arteries when the heart is resting between beats. Think of the diastolic number as measuring the pressure in your arteries when the garden hose is turned off. So if your blood pressure is 140/70, it means that your blood is exerting 140 pounds of pressure against your artery walls when your heart contracts and 70 pounds of pressure when your heart rests. Normal blood pressure is around 120/80.

High Blood Pressure Most doctors would consider regular blood pressure readings over about 140/90 to be high. About 1 in 6 Americans have high blood pressure. But only half of those know they have it.

High blood pressure has been called the silent disease since it very often has no symptoms. However, over time the excessive force exerted on the artery walls may damage the arteries, kidneys, heart and brain, leading to heart attack or stroke.

The specific cause of high blood pressure is not known. But doctors know what makes it worse. Too much salt in the diet, being overweight, lack of exercise and emotional stress may worsen the situation.

Diagnosing High Blood Pressure High blood pressure must be diagnosed over a period of time by taking regular readings. Everyone goes through blood pressure swings throughout the day. It is not uncommon for blood pressure counts to have a 30-point variance in a short period of time. Because of this, high blood pressure can be difficult to diagnose.

Having your blood pressure taken at the doctor's office can often make your blood pressure soar and lead to an incorrect diagnosis, says Bill Sanders of the National Heart, Lung and Blood Institute. This is commonly called the "white coat" syndrome, where a patient gets very anxious in a doctor's office while getting a physical examination. Be sure any diagnosis of high blood pressure is based on a series of readings over time.

Calcium According to a study published in the American Journal of Clinical Nutrition, high blood pressure was reduced in women who took regular calcium supplements. All of the women were taking high blood pressure medication. By supplementing their diet with calcium for a year, blood pressure readings--especially the higher systolic pressure--were reduced significantly. Other women who had normal blood pressure and who supplemented their diet with calcium showed no change in their blood pressure. Women having elevated blood pressure should consider supplementing their diet with about 1,000 mg. of calcium daily.

Fiber A high-fiber diet can lower blood pressure by about 10 percent, says Dr. James Anderson, Professor of Medicine and Clinical Nutrition at the University of Kentucky. After examining the effects of fiber on blood pressure and cholesterol levels on hundreds of patients for ten years, it was found that fiber such as oats, beans and other vegetables, lowers blood pressure (and cholesterol).

Bio-Feed Back Dr. Alan Jacobson of the University of Miami School of Medicine, says that bio-feed back can lower blood pressure. Basically, there are three stages of bio-feed back training:

- The patient is hooked up to a machine that measures the level of muscle tension, letting him see the degree of tension on the bio-feed back machine.
- The machine tells the patient when muscle tension drops or increases. In this way the patient is able to see how tense muscles elevate blood pressure. The patient is then taught how to calm the tense muscles to keep blood pressure under control. Bio-feed back training has helped hundreds of people suffering from high blood pressure to reduce their levels to normal.

24   Self-diagnosis can be dangerous. If you have a serious health problem, see your doctor promptly.

• To get more information on bio-feed back or to get a referral to a qualified practitioner write: The Bio-Feed Back Society of America, 4301 Owens Street, Wheat Ridge, CO 80033, or call 313-422-8436.

Low-Fat Diet Nathan Pritikin, the famous advocate of the low-fat diet, says that excessive fat in the diet is the main cause of high blood pressure. He believes that fat and oil intake cause red blood cells to bunch up and stick together. These clumps of blood cells are unable to pass through the smaller vessels of the circulatory system, acting as "little corks" blocking circulation at thousands of locations throughout the body. When this happens pressure of the blood flowing in the body becomes elevated. With a low-fat diet the blood cells become "un-clumped". The circulatory system expands and pressure drops.

In his two books "The Pritikin Promise" and "The Pritikin Program For Diet and Exercise", Nathan Pritikin documents dozens of cases where persons suffering high blood pressure were able to significantly reduce blood pressure readings and get off blood pressure medication.

Regular Checkups High blood pressure may develop suddenly and without warning. Unless you have regular checkups you may have elevated blood pressure for years without knowing it. High blood pressure is treatable with medication or simple life style changes. Have your blood pressure checked regularly.

BLOWING YOUR NOSE

The Proper Way To Blow Nose There is a proper way to blow your nose to avoid problems with your ear drums. Blow your nose gently, keeping mouth open. If both nostrils are clogged, blow them at the same time, keeping your mouth open. Do not blow each nostril separately.

BODY ODOR

5 Tips To Get Rid Of Body odor is caused by the interaction of bacteria and sweat. Many people suffer body odor despite good personal hygiene. This can cause serious social problems. These recommendations may help avoid body odor:

• Magnesium taken together with zinc, paba and vitamin B-6 can control offensive body odors, according to Dr. B. F. Hart, a physician practicing in Ft. Lauderdale, Florida.

• Don't bathe every day with soap and water. Twice a week is sufficient. Daily bathing washes away natural body oils that lubricate and protect skin from bacteria.

• Use an antibiotic ointment (neomycin solution 0.5 percent) under arms daily after washing.

• Bathe rectal and genital areas and feet daily.

• Don't use commercial deodorants that prevent perspiration. They stop waste products from leaving the body.

BOILS

5 Home Care Suggestions Boils are caused by staphylococci bacteria that enter the skin through a hair follicle. It develops into a pus-filled pocket that comes to a head and finally drains.

• Never squeeze a boil. Most boils rupture and heal on their own. Squeezing may force infection into the blood stream.

• Apply moist heat. Hold a soft cloth soaked with warm water on the boil for 15 minutes, 4 times a day. This will hasten draining.

• The bacteria in the boil is contagious. Disinfect the cloth by boiling or washing in hot water.

• When boil ruptures wash affected area thoroughly and cover with an antibiotic cream and gauze.

• Boils near nose or ears or accompanied by fever should be examined by a doctor promptly.

Zinc For Boil Flareups Supplementing the diet with zinc may help stop boils. Dr. Isser Brody of Sweden noticed that 15 of his patients with a cronic boil problem had low blood levels of zinc. He gave 8 of the patients 45 milligrams of zinc, 3 times a day for about 3 months. Blood zinc levels rose to normal and no new boils occurred. The other 7 patients did not take zinc and continued to suffer recurring boils.

Foods high in zinc include liver, meats, turkey, soybeans, seafood and whole grains.

BREAST CANCER

Minimizing Chance Of Problems Breast cancer is most common in women between the ages of 44 and 55. It is linked to people who are overweight and eat a high fat diet. Breast cancer is treatable if detected early. Over 65% of the victims are still alive after 5 years.

Symptoms Of Breast Cancer
• A lump or thickness with persistant soreness.
• A discharge from the nipple.
• A lump in the armpit.
• Any sensitive area in the breast.
• Any change in skin color or texture especially redness accompanying itching and dimpling of the skin.

Risk Factors Women having the highest risk factors fall into the following categories.

• Women over 40.
• A family history of cancer in females (mother, grandmother, sister, aunt).
• Prior history of benign tumors or other cancer.
• Little sexual activity.

27

- No pregnancies or having a child after age 35.
- Mothers who did not nurse their babies.
- Long term estrogen users or users of oral contraceptives.
- Obesity.
- Living in a highly industrialized area of the U.S.

Preventative Measures
- Read the section of this book under Cancer Risk for information published by the American Institute for Cancer Research on how you can lower your chances of getting cancer.
- Have an annual checkup, especially if you are in a high risk catagory.
- Avoid estrogen therapy.
- Lose weight if you need to.
- Do not smoke.
- Reduce the caffeine in your diet.
- Do a monthly self breast examination.

Breast Self-Examination According to the National Institutes of Health, breast self-examination should be done once a month so you become familiar with the usual appearance and feel of your breasts. Familiarity makes it easier to notice any changes in the breast from one month to another. Early discovery of a change from what is "normal" is the main idea behind Breast Self-Examination.

The National Institutes of Health recommend the following breast self-examination:

1. Stand before a mirror. Inspect both breasts for anything unusual, such as any discharge from the nipples, puckering, dimpling, or scaling of the skin.

2. Watching closely in the mirror, clasp hands behind your head and press hands forward.

3. Next, press hands firmly on hips and bow slightly toward your mirror as you pull your shoulders and elbows forward.

4. Raise your left arm. Use three or four fingers of your

right hand to explore your left breast firmly, carefully and thoroughly. Beginning at the outer edge, press the flat part of your fingers in small circles, moving the circles slowly around the breast. Gradually work toward the nipple. Be sure to cover the entire breast. Pay special attention to the area between the breast and the armpit, including the armpit itself. Feel for any unusual lump or mass under the skin.

5. Gently squeeze the nipple and look for a discharge. Repeat the exam on your right breast.

BRONCHITIS

Supplementing Medical Care Bronchitis is an inflamation of the bronchial tubes. It may be caused by a viral or bacterial infection. Many persons get bronchitis time and again.

• *Vitamin A.* (7500 IU's daily) may help medical treatment by stimulating the mucous membrane upper respiratory tract to resist infections. Foods rich in vitamin A include broccoli, carrots, fish, green and yellow fruits and low-fat milk.

• *Vitamin C.* (500 to 1000 milligrams a day) may increase resistance to bacterial or viral infections. Foods rich in vitamin C include citrus fruits and fruit juices, berries, cabbage, green vegetables and potatoes.

BRUISES

Avoiding Bruises Bruises are caused from breaks in the small blood vessels in the soft tissues beneath the skin. These breaks leak blood which cause a reddish mark on the surface of the skin. This bruise mark turns bluish then yellowish as the blood leak is gradually absorbed.

Vitamin C Several research studies have shown that vitamin C helps strengthen the capillary walls. People who bruise easily can often prevent many bruises by supplementing their diet with vitamin C. Foods rich in vitamin C include citrus fruits and fruit juices, berries, cabbage, green vegetables and potatoes.

Zinc People having low zinc levels were found to bruise easily, according to clinical research studies. Dr. Dean Edell, a prominent San Diego physician, recommends taking 30 mg. of zinc daily if you bruise easily.

BUG BITES

Simple Home Remedy Rubbing meat tenderizer dampened with water on insect bites and stings reduces inflamation and stops pain, says Dr. Paul Drusinski of the University of Vermont.

BURNED TONGUE

How To Relieve Sprinkle a few grains of sugar on the tongue burn. Reapply as necessary. Pain should subside in minutes.

BURNS

First Degree Burns A first degree burn results in damage to the outer layer of the skin only. Some common first degree burns: sunburn, contact with hot objects, hot water or steam.

Symptoms
- Redness.
- Mild swelling.
- Pain.
- Unbroken skin with no blisters.

What To Do. Place the burned area under cold, running water and apply cold water compress such as a clean towel or wash cloth. Do this until pain subsides. Cover the burn with clean bandages. Do not apply butter or grease to a burn. Do not apply other medications without a doctor's recommendation.

Second Degree Burns This is a burn that causes injury to skin beneath the surface of the body. Some common second degree burns include deep sunburn, hot liquids and burns from gasoline and other substances.

Symptoms
- Redness or blotchy appearance to burn.
- Blisters.
- Swelling lasting several days.
- Moist, oozing appearance to the surface of the skin.
- Pain.

What To Do
- Place burned area under cold water (not iced) or apply cold compresses such as a clean towel or wash cloth until pain subsides.
- Gently pat area with dry towel or other soft material.
- Cover burned area with a dry sterile bandage or clean cloth to prevent infection.
- Elevate burned arms or legs.
- Seek medical attention.

Third Degree Burns This kind of burn destroys all layers of the skin. Common third degree burns include prolonged contact with fire, hot substances or electrical burns.

Symtoms
- Burned area is white or charred.
- Skin is destroyed.
- There is little pain because nerve endings have been destroyed.

What To Do
- Do not remove clothes that are stuck to burn.
- Do not put ice or water on burns.
- Do not apply ointment, sprays or antiseptics.
- Consult a doctor immediately

4 Tips For Preventing Burns
- Never smoke in bed or when drowsy.
- When cooking, don't wear loosely fitting, flammable clothing. Bathrobes, nightgowns, and pajamas can catch fire.
- Set water heater thermostats or faucets so that water does not scald the skin.
- Plan which emergency exits to use in case of fire.

BURSITIS

Relieving Pain This is a pain caused by inflamation in the bursae--the small sacs located at the ends of the bones in the joints. These sacs contain lubricating fluids that eliminate friction. The inflamation can result from a sudden pressure or prolonged strain. Common areas of bursitis are the shoulder, elbow, hip, knee and ankle. Tips for easing pain:

- Rest the area affected.
- Apply ice to the painful area three or four times a day for up to 20 minutes at a time.
- After about two days replace the ice treatment with heat treatments. Heat treatments can be with hot packs or heating pads. Or simply take a hot shower. If the pain continues consult a physician.

CALORIES USED

The following list shows the calories used per hour for various kinds of daily activities.

Dancing	330
Bicycling at 5½ miles per hour	210
Bowling	264
Desk work	408
Driving a car	168
Gardening	220
Golf	300
Handball	612
Horseback riding	480
Mowing the lawn	462
Cooking a meal	198
Rollerskating	350
Running at 10 miles per hour	900
Sitting and eating	84
Skiing	594
Sleeping	60
Swimming	300
Tennis	350
Volleyball	350
Walking at 2½ miles per hour	216

CANCER RISK

Cancer On The Increase The American Cancer Society says the number of people expected to get cancer is up--from 1 in 4 for those born in 1970 to 1 in 3 for those born in 1985.

One reason: longer lives increases the risk of cancer. Cancer is the second major cause of death in the U.S. after heart disease.

Lowering The Risk Of Cancer Substantial scientific evidence shows that many cancers are linked to the foods we eat. By eating the right kinds of foods you can reduce the risk of cancer. The American Institute for Cancer Research has published dietary guidelines for lowering the risks of cancer. Here is what the institute recommends:

1. Reduce the intake of fat, both saturated and unsaturated. Americans currently average about 40% of total calories from fat. This level should be reduced to 30% of total calorie intake.
2. Increase the consumption of fruits, vegetables, and whole grains.
3. Consume less salt-cured, smoked and charcoal broiled foods.
4. Drink alcoholic beverages only in moderation.

Hints For Controlling Fat Intake Fat is a valuable part of our diet. It provides energy and essential fatty acids, vitamin D and E. However, most Americans consume more fat than is necessary.

Research suggests that high fat eating habits are associated with greater risk of cancer. Here are some tips for reducing fat intake:

- Meat is a major source of fat in our diets. Limit the size of meat portions to 6 ounces per day. Choose lean meats rather than meats that are fatty. Limit use of sausage and luncheon meats.
- Trim fat from meat and skin from poultry.
- Substitute low-fat dairy products for those high in fat. Use skim milk instead of whole milk. Use low-fat yogurt or imitation sour cream instead of real sour cream. Try evaporated skim milk in recipes that call for heavy cream. Use low-fat cheeses instead of high-fat cheeses. Low-fat

34

cheeses include cottage cheese, part-skim mozzarella and ricotta. High-fat cheeses include cheddar, cream and swiss.

• Read labels carefully. Non-dairy products labeled no cholesterol may still contain large amounts of fat. Choose foods that are labeled as low-fat or contain low-fat items in the list of ingredients.

• Limit fat in cooking. Bake or broil meat--don't fry. Use a rack in the pan when cooking meats to allow fat to drip out. Poach food in water or broth instead of sauteeing it. Use non-stick pans to eliminate the need for fat in cooking. Steam vegetables quickly instead of cooking them in fat.

• Use only small amounts of regular salad dressing.

• Adjust baked goods recipes by using one-half to three-fourths the amount of fat recommended.

• Nuts and seeds are naturally high in fat. Eat them sparingly.

• Choose low-fat, high-nutrient snacks like fresh fruit, raw vegetables, popcorn and whole grain. Limit intake of potato chips, cold cuts, chocolate and ice cream.

Eat More Whole Grains Whole grains should be eaten several times a day. Below are some ways you can use whole grains.

• Substitute whole wheat flour for all-purpose flour in recipes for baked products.

• Check ingredients on ready made bread to ensure that the first ingredient listed is whole grain.

• Use brown rice in place of white rice for greater nutritional value. One cup of uncooked brown rice cooked in 2 cups of water for 50 minutes yeilds about 4 cups of cooked rice.

• Use barley in soup or as a side dish. Whole grain barley is more nutritious than pearl barley. To serve barley as a side dish bring it to boil in about 3 parts water, then cover and simmer 30 to 50 minutes until the barley is tender and the water is absorbed.

• Bulgar is whole wheat that has been steamed, dried and

cracked for quicker cooking. It is a good substitute for rice or potatoes. Cook bulgar in a covered pan with 2 parts water or stock until tender (15 to 18 minutes) and liquid is absorbed.

• Buckwheat has a hearty flavor and is nutritious. If buckwheat is brown it is already roasted. If it is pale, pan roast it briefly before cooking to bring out flavor. Buckwheat should be steamed in 1½ parts boiling water or stock for 15 to 18 minutes.

• Millet is a light textured, mild flavored grain. It can replace rice in most recipes. It should be steamed in 2½ parts liquid for about 20 minutes.

• For breakfast select cereals that have whole grain products first in the list of ingredients.

• Whole grain foods like popcorn or low-fat crackers are excellent snacks that provide more nutrients and fewer calories than potato chips or pretzels.

Eat More Foods Rich In Vitamin A And C Consumption of foods high in beta-carotene (which is converted to vitamin A after consumption) and vitamin C has been associated with lower rates of some cancers. Certain fruits and vegetables are the best source of these nutrients. They provide high levels of other vitamins and minerals in addition to beta-carotene and vitamin C. They are also good sources of dietary fiber. Consume them as frequently as possible.

• The best sources of beta-carotene are dark green and deep yellow fruits and vegetables. These fruits include apricots, cantelope, nectarines, papayas and watermellon. Vegetables high in beta-carotenes include broccoli, carrots, sweet potatoes, winter squash, and all dark, leafy vegetables such as spinach and chard.

• Vitamin C rich fruits include cantelope, grapefruit, oranges and strawberries. The best vegetable sources of vitamin C are broccoli, collard and turnip greens, peppers and tomato juice.

• Try eating vegetables raw or cooked quickly by steaming or stir frying. They stay crispier and more flavorful. Less of

Self-diagnosis can be dangerous. If you have a serious health problem, see your doctor promptly.

the nutrients are destroyed with rapid cooking.

• Try salads made of dark greens such as spinach or non-leafy vegetables such as green peppers, carrots, broccoli, tomatoes and cauliflower.

• Marinate cut-up vegetables in a container with lemon juice or vinegar, herbs and spices. Serve them with meals or as snacks.

• Increase the amount of vegetables in meat-vegetable casseroles while decreasing the amount of meat. Remember large amounts of meat are unnecessary and contribute extra fat to the diet.

• Try the natural sweetness of fruit instead of cookies or candy.

• Substitute fruit or vegetable juices for tea, coffee and soda pop.

Hints For Increasing Use Of Legumes Legumes are dried beans and peas. They are a major part of the diet of many foreign countries. Unfortunately, Americans consume these foods infrequently. Legumes can make a valuable contribution to our diets. They are good sources of protein, iron, magnesium, zinc and several B vitamins. They are high in dietary fiber. For these reasons many health professionals are encouraging increased consumption of legumes.

• Dried beans (kidney, pinto, navy, etc. and lentils) can be combined with other ingredients in soups, salads and stews. They can also be served alone, flavored with herbs and other seasonings. Many people like them pureed and made into sandwich spreads and dips. Tofu (soybean curd) can be cut into cubes and substituted for all or part of the chicken in many casserole or Oriental recipes.

• Beans may be purchased either canned or dried. For convenience canned beans are fine, but dried beans are even more economical.

• Soaking and cooking. One cup of dried beans, peas or lentils expands to 2 or 2½ cups after cooking. Dried beans must be presoaked using either the overnight or quick method. The overnight method: wash beans and place in 4 parts water, cover and let stand 8 hours. Quick method: bring water and beans to a boil and cook for 2 minutes. Cover, remove from heat and let stand for 1 hour. After pre-soaking by either method boil beans gently for 1½ to 2 hours until soft. If you use a pressure cooker, beans can be cooked in 3 to 10 minutes after pre-soaking or in 25 to 45 minutes without pre-soaking.

Be sure to follow package directions carefully because cooking times may vary with the type of beans. Lentils do not need pre-soaking and cook in 30 minutes. If salt is added don't use it until the beans are nearly tender. Salt toughens bean skins and slows cooking. Cooked beans can be stored in the refrigerator for one week or in the freezer for several months.

National Cancer Institute Suggestions For Lowering Cancer Risk

- Don't smoke cigarettes, pipes or cigars. Don't chew tobacco or use snuff.
- Avoid too much sunlight, particularly if you are fair skinned. Use sunscreens and wear protective clothing.
- Don't ask for an x-ray if your doctor or dentist does not recommend it. If you need an x-ray be sure x-ray shields are used to protect other parts of your body.
- If you are exposed to workplace carcinogens, reduce exposure by wearing proper safety clothing.

Colon Cancer: Reducing The Risk Results of a 20-year study published in the medical journal Lancet showed that a diet rich in calcium and vitamin D may help reduce the risk of colon cancer.

The study involved almost 2,000 men. Those men consuming ample amounts of calcium and vitamin D in their diets had almost two-thirds less colon cancer than men consuming low amounts of these nutrients.

Preliminary findings show that consuming about 1,200 milligrams of calcium and about 350 international units

(I.U.'s) of vitamin D each day may significantly cut the risk of colon cancer.

Drinking an 8-ounce glass of skim milk, 4 times a day provides ample amounts of calcium and vitamin D. Other good sources of these nutrients include cottage cheese, low-fat yogurt, salmon and broccoli.

Cancer Information Hotline This toll-free telephone number puts you in contact with a trained specialist who can give personalized answers to questions about cancer causes, prevention, diagnosis and treatment, Call 1-800-4-CANCER.

CANKER SORES

Helpful Suggestions To Stop Flareups Experts say that as many as 50 percent of all Americans suffer canker sores. Canker sores are shallow open sores in the mouth. The inside of the sore is white surrounded by a red border. Some people get them regularly--every month or even every week. The sores usually go away in 7 to 14 days and leave no scars. The exact cause of canker sores is unknown. Some researchers believe they are brought about by sensitivity to certain foods or emotional stress. The following tips may help solve canker sore problems:

• *Zinc.* Taking 50 milligrams of zinc daily has been reported to prevent and shorten the duration of canker sores.
• *Vitamin Deficiency.* Studies by the Institute for Dental Research have shown that some people who get canker sores may be deficient in iron, folic acid and vitamin B-12.
• *Acidophilus.* Many people have reported that taking acidophilus capsules several times a day with meals tends to prevent and clear up the canker sores. This friendly bacteria (lactobacillus Acidophilus) is also in yogurt.

• **Tetracycline.** Some doctors prescribe the anti-biotic tetracycline for canker sores. The treatment involves dissolving a capsule in an ounce of warm water and swishing the mixture in the mouth for 10 minutes, repeating several times a day for about 5 days. The tetracycline mixture is somtimes applied with a cotton swab.

• **Myrrh.** Several druggists recommend an herb called myrrh to treat canker sores. It can be purchased in most health food stores and some drug stores in an alcohol solution. Simply apply with a cotton swab. Just touch the center of the sore. The soreness should subside and healing should follow.

• **Silver Nitrate.** Treating canker sores with silver nitrate shortens the course of the sore, says Dr. John E. Eichenlaub. Simply moisten the tip of a cotton swab with 10% silver nitrate solution (available at any drug store without a prescription). Hold the swab on the canker sore for 5 to 10 seconds then rinse with a little water. After that, wash mouth thoroughly with a mild salt solution 3 or 4 times a day (half a teaspoon of salt in a glass of warm water).

• **Food Allergy.** Many doctors believe canker sores are caused by an allergic reaction to food. Dr. C. W. M. Wilson, from Dublin, Ireland, noticed that most people who suffer canker sores are also allergic to certain foods. The foods most often causing canker sores are coffee, tea, wheat germ, pork, turnips, cabbage, eggs and milk. Dr. Wilson believes the burning and tangy sensations preceeding the canker sore signals consumption of an allergic food. Other foods associated with canker sore flare-ups include citrus fruits and walnuts.

• **Use Soft Tooth Brush.** An experiment on a group of patients experiencing occasional canker sores showed that when pin pricks were made in their mouth canker sores formed where the pin pricks were made. Use a soft tooth brush to avoid any scratching or other trauma to the mouth while brushing your teeth. This alone can significantly alleviate canker sore problems.

CAUSES OF DEATH

10 Worst Killers Of Americans The ten leading causes of death in the United States are as follows:

1. Heart disease
2. Cancer
3. Stroke
4. Accidents
5. Lung Disease
6. Pneumonia and influenza
7. Diabetes
8. Cirrhosis of the liver
9. Circulatory disease
10. Suicide

Most major causes of death are closely associated with diet--especially cancer, heart disease and stroke. Most lung disease is caused by excessive cigarette smoking. Cirrhosis of the liver is mostly caused by excessive alcohol consumption.

CELLULITE

Just Plain Fat Cellulite are those bumpy, cottage cheese-like globs of fat that are around your thighs and stomach. These ugly, orange-peel pits and dimples are just fat, according to Dr. Neil Solomon of Johns-Hopkins University in Baltimore, Maryland.

• Dr. Solomon took samples of cellulite and fat. He found no difference whatsoever in the cells of each. Cellulite and fat are exactly the same.
• Fat and cellulite occur on the body for the same reasons. Excess calories are not burned off and turn to fat.
• The only way to get rid of cellulite is through diet and exercise.

CHAFING

Tips For Relieving Chafing
● Apply hydrocortisone creme sparingly, twice a day for 3 to 4 days.
● Apply zinc oxide ointment twice a day, then clean it off with baby or mineral oil.
● Applying baby powder to the skin may protect sensitive areas from chafing.

CHOKING

What To Do When You're Alone
● When you start to choke make a fist with the thumb curled outside.
● Place your fist, thumb side, against your abdomen slightly above the naval and below the rib cage.
● Then grasp your fist with your free hand and press it into your abdomen with a quick upper thrust.
● Repeat the maneuver until the foreign object is expelled. This is called the Heimlich maneuver developed by Dr. Henry Heimlich. You can perform the maneuver standing, sitting or even lying down.

CHOLESTEROL (See Also HEART DISEASE)

Cause Of Heart Disease And Stroke Cholesterol is a fat-like, pearly substance found in saturated animal fats and oils. Foods high in cholesterol include egg yolks, cream, butter, cheese and fatty meats. The normal blood cholesterol level ranges from 150 to 250 milligrams per deciliter (1/10th of a quart). Many specialists recommend keeping cholesterol levels below 200. Some specialists recommend keeping it under 150.

Many studies have shown that high cholesterol levels increase your risk of heart attack and stroke. Here's how doctors say cholesterol damages your body: Cholesterol is carried in the blood stream where some is deposited in the inner linings of the arteries. These fatty deposits build up causing the artery walls to thicken and become less flexible. The artery narrows and restricts blood flow. Eventually, the blood supply may be shut off completely. If the blood stoppage is in an artery feeding the brain a stroke may result. If the clogged artery feeds the heart, a heart attack may occur.

Reducing Cholesterol In Your Diet

- Choose lean meat, fish, poultry, dried beans and peas as protein sources.
- Moderate use of eggs and organ meats such as liver and kidneys.
- Use skim or low fat milk.
- Limit intake of butter, cream, shortenings, coconut oil and foods made from such products.
- Eat less sausage, bacon and processed luncheon meats.
- Trim excess fat off meats.
- Broil, bake and boil rather than fry.
- Read labels carefully to determine amounts and type of fat in foods.

Fat In Your Diet--Saturated and Unsaturated Saturated fat is usually hard at room temperature. For example, fat on cooked beef becomes hard and white if left out at room temperature. The major sources of saturated fat in our diet is meat and dairy products. Saturated fat intake is a strong contributor to raising blood cholesterol levels.

Polyunsaturated fat stays soft or in liquid form at room temperature. All vegetable oils are rich in polyunsaturated fat

43

and have no cholesterol. Polyunsaturated fat will lower blood cholesterol, according to the National Heart, Lung and Blood Institute.

The chart below shows the percent of polyunsaturated fat and staurated fat for various types of oil or fat. When you use oils or fats choose those high in polyunsaturated fat--the ones at the top of the chart--according to the National Institutes of Health.

Type of Oil or Fat	Percent Polyunsaturated Fat	Percent Saturated Fat
Safflower Oil	74%	9%
Sunflower Oil	64%	10%
Corn Oil	58%	13%
Average Vegetable Oil (soybean plus cottonseed)	40%	13%
Peanut Oil	30%	19%
Chicken Fat (Schmaltz)	26%	29%
Olive Oil	9%	14%
Average Vegetable Shortening	20%	32%
Lard	12%	40%
Beef Fat	4%	48%
Butter	4%	61%
Palm Oil	2%	81%
Coconut Oil	2%	86%

Self-diagnosis can be dangerous. If you have a serious health problem, see your doctor promptly.

When You're At Risk

Cholesterol
(in milligrams per deciliter)

Age	Moderate Risk	High Risk
2-19	Over 170	Over 185
20-29	Over 200	Over 220
30-39	Over 220	Over 240
40 and up	Over 240	Over 260

Source: National Institutes of Health consensus conference statement, Lowering Blood Cholesterol, 1984.

COCAINE USERS HELP HOTLINE

Call Toll-Free For Help This is a little-known, free service provided by the Federal government. Hotline operators provide information on coping with drug related problems. The line is open to users and concerned relatives and friends. They can refer abusers to professional help. 1-800-COCAINE.

COFFEE

Greater Risk Of Heart Attack A Stanford University study showed that coffee increases the level of certain types of cholesterol in the blood. Men drinking 2 cups of coffee or more a day face a higher risk of heart disease. Coffee should be drunk only in moderation, say researchers.

COLD (COMMON)

Try Zinc To Shorten Misery Zinc can reduce the time you will be affected by a common cold, says Dr. Jeffrey Fisher, Medical Director of the Extensis Medical Center in Roslyn, New York. Zinc appears to kill the viruses that cause the common cold. Zinc won't prevent a cold, but it can stimulate the body's infection-fighting defenses--thus reducing the time a cold will make you miserable.

- Zinc was tested on 65 volunteers suffering from colds. Thirty-seven were given zinc. Those individuals suffered only 3.7 days. The other volunteers were given a fake pill. They suffered an average of 10.8 days--almost 3 times longer.
- The dosage of zinc was 23 milligrams of zinc (gluconate) every 2 hours with a maximum dosage of 12 tablets or 250 milligrams.
- The zinc tablets should not be swallowed. They have to be sucked over a period of about 10 minutes.
- The zinc should not be taken for more than one week. It may upset the balance of copper in your system and upset the immune system.
- Pre-sweetened lozenges available at most health food stores are recommended. If not available suck zinc tablets along with a sweet mint to mask the zinc taste. Consult your physician before taking zinc supplements.

Vitamin C Vitamin C may help shorten the duration of a common cold, according to a study published in the Medical Journal of Australia. The study involved 95 pairs of twins. One pair of twins took 100 milligrams of vitamin C for 100 days. The other twins took a fake pill. Twins taking the vitamin C recovered from cold symptoms 19% sooner. Foods rich in vitamin C include citrus fruits, fruit juices, berries, cabbage, green vegetables and potatoes.

Other Helpful Suggestions
- Stay in bed if possible.

- Take aspirin or acetaminophen (like Tylenol). Don't take aspirin with vitamin C. The combination may increase stomach irritation.
- Do not smoke--stay away from others who do smoke. Cigarette smoking weakens resistence and lung power.
- Avoid complications by staying away from crowds.
- Eat properly and consult your doctor if condition worsens.

COLD SORES (FEVER BLISTERS)

Home Remedies Cold sores are caused by the herpes simplex virus. This virus affects about 85% of the U.S. population. Some doctors believe it is the second most common ailment--next to the common cold.

The cold sore starts as a tiny, painful red spot generally on the lip or corner of the mouth. These sores form a blister that turns into a scab. This scab lasts from 7 to 14 days. Many people regularly suffer cold sores. Cold sores can be transmitted by hugging, kissing and other direct contact. Try these suggestions for cold sore relief:

- *Vitamin E.* Dr. Don Nead, a dentist from Redding, California, uses vitamin E to treat cold sores. He recommends applying 20,000 IU's for about 15 minutes, 3 times a day. This relieves or eliminates cold sore pain in less than 8 hours. The sore actually heals itself in 12 to 24 hours in many cases. Dr. Nead reports an almost 100% success rate with this method.
- *Ice.* This ancient remedy really helps. According to several physicians, cold sores are best treated by holding an ice cube directly on the erupted cold sore for 45 minutes. This is more effective and cheaper than any other drug treatment. One physician said cold sores usually dry up in a day or two after ice cube treatments.

• *Lysine.* Cold sores can also be successfully treated with the amino acid lysine, says Dr. Christopher Kagan of Cedar-Sinai Medical Center in Los Angeles, California. Lysine counteracts the production of the herpes virus, he believes. He conducted a study on 25 persons suffering from recurring cold sores. They were given 800 to 1,000 milligrams of lysine each day. The patients reported less pain, faster healing and less frequent recurrence of the cold sores. Lysine is available at health food stores.

In another study, researchers at Indiana University gave lysine to 250 patients suffering cold sores. The dosage ranged from 312 to 1200 milligrams daily. Only 2 percent of the subjects showed no improvement. Researchers say if lysine is taken at first sign of stinging pain an attack may be averted.

• *Yogurt.* Dr. Morton Malkin, a dentist from Brooklyn, New York, recommends yogurt for cold sores. Yogurt contains lactobacillus acidophilus (or lactobacillus bulgaricus). The doctor believes these good bacteria crowd out the herpes cold sores in the body. He also recommends high doses of vitamin B-complex and increased fluid intake. Hundreds of patients have been treated with this method.

COMPUTER EYE STRAIN

Tips To Avoid Eye strain caused by using a computer is very common, causing symptoms such as headache, blurred vision and burning eyes, says Dr. R. Anthony Hutchinson of San Diego, California. Follow these rules to avoid problems:

• Position yourself about 22 inches from the screen.
• Get rid of glare reflecting off your computer screen.
• Blink your eyes periodically.
• Take scheduled breaks from the computer.
• Have your eyes examined to make sure you do not need glasses. Make sure you have the proper prescription.

CONSTIPATION

Conditions That Can Cause It is not necessary to have a bowel movement every day. From 3 bowel movements each day to 3 each week is considered normal. Constipation can be accompanied by fatigue, headache, bloatiness and mild cramps. The following can cause constipation:

• Diets low in fiber or roughage and high in animal fat can cause constipation.

• Stress can lead to constipation. Also certain drugs, including antacids and pain relievers, can cause problems.

• Travel can cause constipation. This is due to changes in drinking water, diet and daily activities.

• Older people sometimes suffer constipation because of not drinking enough fluids, lack of exercise and low fiber diets.

• Pregnancy can cause constipation.

• Over-use of laxatives resulting in dependence is a common cause of constipation.

Suggestions For Avoiding Constipation

• Eat fruit, raw vegetables, bran, high bulk foods, whole grain bread and whole grain cereals.

• Eat regularly.

• Get plenty of physical exercise.

• Drink a half glass of hot water one-half hour before breakfast every day. Drink a total of 8 glasses of fluids daily-- two should be prune juice.

• Never strain. Be relaxed.

• Have regular bowel movements at the same time of day. The best time is a half hour or so after breakfast.

• If you're still having difficulty add an ounce of mineral oil to fruit juice and drink before retiring.

Try Yogurt and Prunes A study published in the Journal of the American Medical Association showed that a mixture of yogurt and prunes helps constipation. The study involved

194 patients suffering constipation. Nearly all the participants experienced relief by taking a mixture of yogurt and prunes. Researchers believe the lactobacillus acidophilus in yogurt helps promote regularity.

CONTACT LENSES

Common Problems With Contact Lenses
• *Bacterial Infection.* If the infection is serious it can leave scars on your eye and decrease vision. The most common cause of infection is poor hygiene--especially when surface of cornia is scratched, says Dr. R. Linsy Farris.

• *Scratches.* Scratched cornia on inner eyelid can also turn to infection.

• *Allergic Reactions.* This can be caused by chemicals used to clean the lenses.

• *Discomfort.* Pain can result from abrasions on the cornia caused by wearing hard contact lenses too long.

Protecting Yourself From Injury
• Make sure you are examined by a qualified eye doctor.
• Have regular follow-up examinations.
• Be sure you understand how to insert and remove your lenses.
• Learn proper hygiene techniques from your doctor.

CONTRACEPTIVES

Comparing The Options A number of contraception methods are available today. Some can be obtained without a doctor's prescription or advice. Others require a prescription, medical consultation and followup.

Basic information on the contraceptive methods most

widely used is explained below. This is only beginning information to help you understand the choices available. Discussion with a physician can help you make a selection that is right for you.

No method of contraception is 100 percent effective. Correct use of a method is essential to ensure maximum effectiveness. The more care taken in using a method exactly as instructed, the more effective it will be. Using a combination of methods (such as diaphragm and condom, foam and condom, etc.) also will increase the contraceptive effectiveness.

The Pill "The Pill" refers to any of the oral contraceptives. The most widely used contains two female hormones, estrogen and progestin--taken 21 days each month. Another (sometimes called the "mini-pill") contains progestin only and is taken continuously. You should receive from the druggist, doctor or person who gives you the pills an FDA-required brochure explaining the use, benefits and risks of the product in greater detail.

Effectiveness of The Pill
- Effectiveness depends on how correctly the method is used. Of 100 women who use the combination estrogen and progestin pill for one year, less than 1 will become pregnant. Of 100 women who use the progestin-only pill (mini-pill) for one year, 2 to 3 will become pregnant.

Advantages
- The combination pill is the most effective of all popular methods of preventing pregnancy.
- No inconvenient devices to bother with at time of intercourse.

Disadvantages
- Must be taken regularly and exactly as instructed by the prescribing physician.

Side Effects
- Side effects may include tender breasts, nausea, vomiting,

51

gain or loss of weight, unexpected vaginal bleeding, higher levels of sugar and fat in the blood.

• Although it happens infrequently, use of the Pill can cause blood clots (in the legs, and less frequently in the lungs, brain and heart). A clot that reaches the lungs or forms in the brain or heart can be fatal. Pill users have a greater risk of heart attack and stroke than non-users. This risk increases with age and is greater if the Pill user smokes.

• Some Pill users tend to develop high blood pressure. It usually is mild and may by reversed by discontinuing use.

• Pill users have a greater risk than non-users of having gallbladder disease requiring surgery.

• There is no substantial evidence that taking the Pill increases the risk of cancer. Rarely, benign liver tumors occur in women on the Pill. Sometimes they rupture, causing fatal hemorrhage.

Health Factors to Consider

• Women who use the Pill are strongly advised not to smoke because smoking increases the risk of heart attack or stroke.

• Other women who should not take the Pill are those who have had a heart attack, stroke, angina pectoris, blood clots, cancer of the breast or uterus. Women who have scanty or irregular periods should be encouraged to use some other method.

• A woman who believes she may be pregnant should not take the Pill because it increases the risk of defect in the fetus.

• Health problems, such as migraine headaches, mental depression, fibroids of the uterus, heart or kidney disease, asthma, high blood pressure, diabetes, or epilepsy may be made worse by use of the Pill.

• Risks associated with the Pill increase with age.

Long-Term Effect on Ability to Have Children

• There is no evidence that using the Pill will prevent a woman from becoming pregnant after she stops taking it, although there may be a delay before she is able to become pregnant. Women should wait a short time after stopping the Pill before becoming pregnant. During this time another method of contraception should be used.

● After childbirth the woman should consult her doctor before resuming use of the Pill. This is especially true for nursing mothers. The drugs in the Pill appear in the milk and the long-range effect on the infant is not known.

Intrauterine Device (IUD) The IUD is a small plastic or metal device that is placed in the uterus (womb) through the cervical canal (opening into the uterus). As long as the IUD stays in place pregnancy is prevented. How the IUD prevents pregnancy is not completely understood. IUD's seem to interfere in some manner with implantation of the fertilized egg in the wall of the uterus. There are 5 kinds of IUD's currently available--Copper-7, Copper-T, Progestasert, Lippes Loop, and Saf-T-Coil. IUD's containing copper (Copper-7 and Copper-T) should be replaced every 3 years. Those containing progesterone (Progestasert) should be replaced every year.

Effectiveness
● Effectiveness depends on proper insertion by the physician and whether the IUD remains in place.
● Of 100 women who use an IUD for one year, 1 to 6 will become pregnant.

Advantages
● Insertion by a physician, then no further care needed, except to see that the IUD remains in place (the user can check it herself but should be checked once a year by her doctor).

Disadvantages
● May cause pain or discomfort when inserted. Afterward may cause cramps and a heavier menstrual flow. Some women will experience adverse effects that require removal of the IUD.

Self-diagnosis can be dangerous. If you have a serious health problem, see your doctor promptly.

53

• The IUD can be expelled, sometimes without being aware of it, leaving you unprotected.

Side Effects
• Major complications, which are infrequent, include anemia, pregnancy outside the uterus, pelvic infection, perforation of the uterus or cervix, and septic abortion.

• A woman with heavy or irregular bleeding while using an IUD should consult her physician. Removal of the IUD may be necessary to prevent anemia.

• Women susceptible to pelvic infection are more prone to infection when using an IUD.

• Serious complications can occur if a woman becomes pregnant while using an IUD. Though rare, cases of blood poisoning, miscarriage, and even death have been reported. An IUD user who believes she may be pregnant should consult her doctor immediately. If pregnancy is confirmed, the IUD should be removed.

• Although it rarely happens, the IUD can pierce the wall of the uterus when it is being inserted. Surgery is required to remove it.

Health Factors to Consider
• Before having an IUD inserted, you should tell your doctor of any of the following: cancer or other abnormalities of the uterus or cervix; bleeding between periods or heavy menstrual flow; infection of the uterus, cervix, or pelvis (pus in fallopian tubes); prior IUD use; recent pregnancy, abortion, or miscarriage; uterine surgery; venereal disease; severe menstrual cramps; allergy to copper; anemia; fainting attacks; unexplained genital bleeding or vaginal discharge; suspicious or abnormal "Pap" smear.

Long-Term Effect on Having Children
• Pelvic infection in some IUD users may result in their future inability to have children.

Diaphragm (With Cream, Jelly or Foam) A diaphragm is a shallow cup of thin rubber stretched over a flexible ring. A sperm-killing cream or jelly is put on both sides of the diaphragm, which is then placed inside the vagina before intercourse. The device covers the opening of the uterus, thus preventing the sperm from entering the uterus.

Effectiveness
• Effectiveness depends on how correctly the method is used. Of 100 women who use the diaphragm with a spermicidal product for one year, 2 to 20 will become pregnant.

Advantages
• No routine schedule to be kept as with the Pill. The diaphragm with a spermicidal product is inserted by the user.
• No discomfort or cramping, as with the IUD. No effect on the chemical or physical processes of the body, as with the Pill or the IUD.

Disadvantages
• Must be inserted before each intercourse and stay in place 6 to 8 hours afterwards.
• Size and fit require yearly checkup and should be checked if you gain or lose weight.
• Should be refitted after childbirth or abortion.
• Requires instruction on insertion technique. Some women find it difficult to insert and inconvenient to use.
• Some women having a greatly relaxed vagina or "fallen" uterus cannot use a diaphragm successfully.

Side Effects
• No serious side effects.
• Possible allergic reaction to the rubber or the spermicidal jelly. Condition easily corrected.

Foam, Cream or Jelly Alone (including Suppositories*) Several brands of vaginal foam, cream or jelly can be used without a diaphragm. They form a chemical barrier at the opening of the uterus that prevents sperm from reaching an egg in the uterus. They also destroy sperm.

Effectiveness
- Effectiveness depends on how correctly the method is used. Of 100 women who use aerosol foams alone for one year, 2 to 29 will become pregnant.
- Of 100 women who use jellies and creams alone for one year, 4 to 36 will become pregnant.
- No figures available for suppositories--considered fair to poor.

Advantages
- Easy to obtain and use. No devices needed.

Disadvantages
- Must be used one hour or less before intercourse. If placed earlier, may become ineffective.
- If douching is desired, must wait 6 to 8 hours after intercourse.

Side Effects
- No serious side effects. Burning or irritation of the vagina or penis may occur. Allergic reaction may be corrected by changing brands.

Female Sterilization The primary method of sterilization for women is tubal sterilization, commonly referred to as "tying the tubes." A surgeon cuts, ties or seals the fallopian tubes to prevent passage of eggs between the ovaries and the uterus. Several techniques are available. With one new technique, the operation can be performed in a hospital outpatient surgical clinic with either a local or general anesthetic. Using this method, the doctor makes a tiny incision in the abdomen or vagina and blocks the tubes by cutting, sealing with an electric current, or applying a small band or clip. Hysterectomy, a surgical procedure involving removal of all or part of the uterus, also prevents pregnancy, but is performed for other medical reasons and is not considered primarily a method of sterilization.

Effectiveness
• Virtually 100 percent.

Advantages
• A one-time procedure--never any more bother with devices or preparations of any kind.

Disadvantages
• Surgery is required. Although in some cases a sterilization procedure has been reversed through surgery, the procedure should be considered permanent.

Side Effects
• As with any surgery, occasionally there are complications, such as severe bleeding, infection or injury to other organs which may require additional surgery to correct.

Health Factors to Consider
• There is some risk associated with any surgical procedure, which varies with the general health of the patient.

Long-Term Effect on Ability to Have Children
• When the traditional type of tubal ligation is used, it is reversible in some cases. However, ability to reverse should not be counted on.

Male Sterilization Sterilization of men involves severing the tubes through which the sperm travel to become part of the semen. The man continues to produce sperm but they are absorbed by the body rather than being released into the semen. This operation, called a vasectomy, takes about half an hour and may be performed in a doctor's office under local anesthetic. A vasectomy does not affect a man's physical ability to have intercourse.

Effectiveness
• Virtually 100 percent.

Advantages
• A one-time procedure that does not require

hospitalization and permits the man to resume normal activity almost immediately.

Disadvantages
• The man is not sterile immediately after the operation-- usually it takes a few months. Other means of contraception must be used during that time.

Side Effects
• Complications occur in 2 to 4 percent of cases, including infection, hematoma (trapped mass of clotted blood), granuloma (an inflammatory reaction to sperm that is absorbed by the body), and swelling and tenderness near the testes. Most such complications are minor and are treatable without surgery.

• Studies by the National Institutes of Health show that vasectomy does not affect a man's sexual desire or ability.

Long-Term Effect on Ability to Have Children
• Male sterilization is reversible in a fair number of cases, but ability to reverse should not be counted on.

Condom (Rubber) The condom is a thin sheath of rubber or processed lamb cecum that fits over the penis.

Effectiveness
• Effectiveness depends on how correctly the method is used. Of 100 women whose partner uses a condom for one year, 3 to 36 women will become pregnant.

Advantages
• In addition to contraception, may provide some protection against venereal disease.

• Easily available. Requires no "long-term" planning before intercourse.

Disadvantages
• Some people feel the condom reduces pleasure in the sex act.

• The male must interrupt foreplay and fit the condom in

place before sexual entry into the woman.

• The condom can slip or tear during use or spill during removal from the vagina.

Side Effects

No serious side effects. Occasionally an individual will be allergic to the rubber, causing burning, irritation, itching, rash, or swelling, but this can easily be treated. Switching to the natural skin condom may be a solution.

Natural Family Planning (Rhythm Method) The woman must refrain from sexual intercourse on days surrounding the predicted time of monthly ovulation or, for greater effectiveness, until a few days after the predicted time of ovulation. Ways to determine the approximate time of ovulation include a calendar method, temperature method, cervical mucus method, and a sympto-thermal method. Using the calendar method requires careful recordkeeping of the time of the menstrual period and calculation of the time in the month when the woman is fertile and must not have intercourse. To use the temperature method, the woman must use a special type of thermometer and keep an accurate daily record of her body temperature (body temperature rises after ovulation). To use the cervical mucus method the woman must keep an accurate daily record of the type of vaginal secretions present. To use the sympto-thermal method the woman must observe the changes in her cervix, cervical mucus, and also record her body temperature every day to pinpoint her fertile period. The temperature method, mucus method, or sympto-thermal method used alone or concurrently with the calendar method are more effective than the calendar method alone.

Effectiveness

• Effectiveness depends on how correctly the method is used. Of 100 women who use the calendar method for one year, 14 to 47 will become pregnant.

• Of 100 women who use the temperature method for one year, 1 to 20 will become pregnant.

- Of 100 women who use the mucus method for one year, 1 to 25 will become pregnant.
- Of 100 women who use, for one year, the temperature or mucus method with intercourse only after ovulation, less than 1 to 7 will become pregnant.
- Of 100 women who use the sympto-thermal method for one year, 1 to 22 will become pregnant.

Advantages
- No drugs or devices needed.

Disadvantages
- Requires careful recordkeeping and estimation of the time each month when there can be no intercourse.
- To use any of the three methods properly a physician's guidance may be needed, at least at the outset.
- If menstrual cycles are irregular, it is especially difficult to use this method effectively.
- Dissatisfaction because of extended time each month when sexual intercourse must be avoided.

Side Effects
- No physical effects, but because the couples must refrain from having intercourse except on certain days of the month, using this method can create pressures on the couple's relationship.

Withdrawal (Coitus Interruptus) This method of contraception requires withdrawal of the male organ (penis) from the vagina before the man ejaculates, so the male sperm are not deposited at or near the birth canal. This method should not be considered effective for preventing pregnancy.

Douching Use of a vaginal douche immediately after sexual intercourse to wash out or inactivate male sperm is not considered effective for preventing pregnancy.

COOLING DOWN IN HOT WEATHER

Follow These Simple Tips
- Reduce calorie intake. Eat less fats and proteins. Eat more carbohydrates such as vegetables and fruits.
- Avoid midday sun.
- Wear light clothing. Light colors are good because they reflect sun. Dark clothing absorbs the sun.
- Drink at least 8 glasses of liquid a day. Water is the best drink. Take time out to drink liquids even if you don't feel thirsty.
- Eating melons is a good way to increase your fluid intake. Watermelons and cantelopes have significant amounts of water.
- Make sure drinks do not have sugar in them.
- Eat small meals rather than large ones. Digestion adds to body heat.
- Replace potassium and salt lost through sweat. Citrus fruit and bananas are good sources of potassium.
- Avoid alcoholic beverages. It acts as a diuretic resulting in faster water loss.
- Take cool showers. Water removes extra body heat 25 times faster than cool air.
- Avoid heavy physical activity.

If Body Temperature Reaches 105 Degrees Fahrenheit (Heat Stroke)
1. Spray victim with hose. Sponge bare skin with cold water or rubbing alcohol. Apply cold packs to the victim's body.
2. Continue treatment until body temperature is lowered to 101 or 102 degrees Fahrenheit.
3. Do not overchill. Check temperature constantly.
4. Dry victim off once temperature is lowered.
5. Seek medical attention quickly, preferrably at the nearest hospital emergency room.

COSMETICS

Little Difference Among Brands Most cosmetics on the market today have similar ingredients, according to reports by the U.S. Food and Drug Administration. This means that expensive products are no more effective than moderately priced ones. With the expensive face cream, the buyer may be paying for an attractive jar or a brand name.

CRABS

What To Do Crabs are tiny insects that infest the pubic hair area. They attach to the base of the hair root. They cause blue spots on the skin and considerable itching.

Crabs can be transmitted through personal contact or sexual intercourse. They can also be acquired from a toilet seat, clothing or sleeping in an infested bed.

Treatment consists of rubbing the affected area with an anti-crab ointment available at the drug store. Some good commercial preparations are Kwell and Cuprex.

DANDRUFF

Controlling Dandruff Dandruff is a mild inflamation of the scalp causing flaking. These flakes are often highly visible on the hair and even fall onto the shoulders. A compound called selenium, found in several drug store shampoo products, is highly effective in controlling dandruff. The shampoo should be left on at least 5 minutes before rinsing thoroughly. The hair and scalp should be shampooed at least once a week.

Vitamins And Minerals Richard Gerson, PhD., in his book "The Right Vitamins", says dandruff may be due to nutritional deficiencies. He recommends getting adequate amounts of vitamin B-6, B-12, F and selenium in your diet.

Peanut Oil And Lemon Many people report relief from dandruff with an old-time remedy combining peanut oil and lemon juice. Simply rub warm peanut oil into your scalp. Then apply the juice from a fresh lemon. Leave on for a few minutes then shampoo your hair. According to Dr. Alan Shalita of the State University of New York Dermatology Department, the old-time remedy has value.

DENTURES

Calcium Helps Living With Dentures Millions of Americans wear dentures. Dentures can often be inconvenient, clumsy and cause considerable pain. A large part of the discomfort of dentures can come from the underlying bone in the gums which shrinks and causes improper fit.

Adding extra calcium to your diet can slow down the bone shrinking process, says Dr. Kenneth Wycal from Loma Linda University. Dr. Wycal studied two groups of denture wearers. One group supplemented their diets with 750 milligrams of calcium plus vitamin D each day. The other group did not supplement their diet. After one year those supplementing their diets with calcium lost an average of 34% less jawbone than the others, making dentures fit better. Foods rich in vitamin D include milk, salmon, tuna and sardines.

DEPRESSION (THE BLUES)

Chasing Away The Blues Depression is a serious problem in America. Doctors estimate that more than 20 million Americans suffer some form of depression.

63

Depression might last for days, weeks or even longer. Women suffer from depression twice as often as men. Many experts believe depression often stems from anger that is not expressed. These held in feelings eventually turn into depression. If depression continues professional help may be needed. The following suggestions may help beat the blues:

● **Minerals May Help.** Calcium and magnesium may help the blues, according to one study published in the Journal of Nervous and Mental Disease. The study showed that depressed patients had significantly lower blood levels of magnesium than healthy people.

Dr. August Daro, a Chicago obstetrician and gynecologist, says he routinely gives his depressed patients calcium and magnesium. He recommends combinations of 400 milligrams of calcium and 200 milligrams of magnesium per day. These minerals calm the nervous system and make depressed people feel better. He also recommends calcium and magnesium for premenstrual depression. Calcium and magnesium are available at most drug stores and health food stores.

● **Low Folic Acid And Depression.** Researchers found that folic acid levels were significantly lower in depressed patients than in patients not suffering from depression, according to a study published in Psychosomatics. Folic acid is part of the vitamin B family. It is crucial to the normal functioning of the central nervous system. Folic acid is available in most health food stores. Foods rich in folic acid include beets, cabbage, green leafy vegetables, citrus fruits and whole grains.

● **Amino Acid--Tyrosine.** A study published in the American Journal of Psychiatry indicated that supplementing the diet with the amino acid tyrosine helped some patients with depression. Of the 11 patients included in the study, 9 showed improvement after taking tyrosine. Tyrosine is available in most health food stores.

● **Low Blood Sugar.** Low blood sugar (hypoglycemia) is a common cause of depression, according to Dr. August Daro, a Chicago medical doctor. When he sees a depressed patient, the first thing he does is give a glucose tolerance test to measure blood sugar levels.

• *Coffee And Depression.* Some doctors believe drinking a lot of coffee can cause anxiety and even depression. Symptoms of anxiety may occur after drinking as few as 2 cups of coffee--about 250 milligrams of caffeine. Cola beverages supply about 40 milligrams per serving. A small chocolate bar, about 25 milligrams. It doesn't take much to reach the 250 milligram level, researchers say.

• *Low Tryptophane Levels.* A study published in the British Medical Journal researched 18 women who suffered from depression. The researchers found that blood levels of tryptophane were low in all 18 women. The amino acid tryptophane is available at most health food stores.

• *Vitamin B-6 And Depression.* Numerous studies have shown that women on the birth control pill may become depressed due to low levels of vitamin B-6. For example, in one study published in the Medical Journal Lancet, doctors measured the blood level of vitamin B-6 in 39 depressed women taking the birth control pill. They found 19 had a severe vitamin B-6 deficiency. When these women were given vitamin B-6, sixteen improved in mood. Foods rich in vitamin B-6 include bananas, cabbage, green leafy vegetables, whole grains and fish.

Another study showed that 15 depressed, pregnant women had low blood levels of vitamin B-6. These women were not taking birth control pills. This study was published in the Acta Obstetricia et Gynecologica Scandinavica.

• *Another Amino Acid May Help.* Researchers found that depressed patients may benefit from an amino acid called phenylalanine, according to a study performed at Queen Charlottes Maternity Hospital in London. Phenylalanine is available in most health food stores.

DIARRHEA

3 Natural Remedies
• *Yogurt.* Many countries use yogurt as a treatment for

diarrhea. The friendly bacteria in yogurt called acidophilus tends to help normalize bowel functions. Yogurt has an antibiotic effect, especially against E. coli, the main cause of traveler's diarrhea.

• *Bran.* Bran helps normalize the bowel function. Bran helps relieve both constipation and diarrhea. Bran thickens the loose stool of diarrhea and softens the hard, dry stools in constipation.

• *Carob Powder.* A Canadian study showed that 227 of 230 infants given carob powder in their formula got relief from diarrhea. Only 3 cases were not helped. Carob contains a high level of fiber.

What To Eat
1. Avoid solid foods.
2. Start a clear liquid diet to replace lost fluids. This would include water, tea, carbonated beverages, jello or broth.
3. If diarrhea lasts longer than a day or two, seek medical attention. Prolonged diarrhea causes dehydration.

DIETING

How To Successfully Lose Weight Obesity is a national health problem. It is estimated that 60 million Americans are above their ideal weight.

The cause of being overweight is nearly always the direct result of eating more food than is burned off by activity. These excess calories are stored in the body as fat. The more calories taken in above what is burned off, the fatter we become. Each 3,500 excess calories equals 1 pound of body fat.

The only way to lose weight is: eat less and exercise more. Low calorie eating habits that are nutritionally well-balanced is the key to successful weight loss. This combined with a regular exercise program should keep weight off permanently. Anyone starting a diet and exercise program should consult a doctor.

Dangers of Obesity Being overweight exposes you to numerous risks and even premature death. Overweight persons are more prone to heart and kidney disease, diabetes, high blood pressure, liver disorders and arthritis. Being 20 pounds overweight between age 40 and 50 increases chance of death 18 percent.

Avoid Crash Diets Crash diets can be dangerous. Losing weight too fast may damage the heart, gastrointestinal trace and metabolism. Rigid dieting and extreme weight fluctuations increase risk of gall stones, according to medical studies.

A study conducted at Case Western University showed that the most successful dieters lost weight at a slow steady pace.

What To Do Before Meals
- Don't let yourself get too hungry before meals.
- Tighten your belt.
- Start a meal with a cup of low-calorie soup.
- Eat a salad 10 or 15 minutes before your meal. This will help cut your appetite down. Of course, eat your salad with a low-calorie dressing.
- Drink a glass of ice water. It has a shrinking effect on the stomach. Helps curb appetite and makes stomach feel fuller, according Dr. Richard Hansen of Poland Spring Health Institute in Maine.
- Drink a large glass of water before each meal. Drink it slowly. Food is more than 50% water. When you crave food you may really be craving water.

During Meals--Suggestions For Successful Dieting
- Eat meals at regular intervals.
- Eat fewer sweets. Substitute artificial sweetners instead.
- Cut down on alcohol intake. Whiskey and beer are high in calories.
- Eat more fiber. Vegetables, fruit, whole grains and beans

add bulk to your diet and make you feel full and satisfied.

• Cut down on fats. Don't fry your foods. Avoid fatty cuts of meat. Trim off all visible fat on your foods. Remove skin from chicken before cooking.

• Eat slowly. People who eat fast often overeat. This is because they eat so fast they don't realize how much they have eaten until it is too late. Try eating with a small cocktail fork.

• Instead of giving up your favorite foods just eat those foods in much smaller quantities.

• Use herbs and spices to flavor food. Avoid high calorie dressings and toppings.

• Take smaller bites and put your fork down after each bite. You'll eat less.

• Put meals on a small plate rather than a large plate.

Stopping The Binging Urge

• When you get the urge to binge put on some of your tight clothes. Experience the discomfort for a few hours. Imagine how good it would feel to wear them without the tightness.

• To satisfy the snack cravings make popsicles using flavored water and low calorie sweeteners.

• When eating at a buffet or party with a wide variety of foods take only tiny servings of each dish.

Try Glucomannan Capsules Preliminary research shows that taking glucomannan capsules before meals increases weight loss. Glucomannan capsules are available in health food stores. Glucomannan is a natural fiber that swells up in the stomach reducing the desire for food.

• A study conducted at Harvard showed that dieters lost twice as much weight on glucomannan capsules. One hundred overweight women were put on a 12-week diet of 1,000 calories a day along with 20 overweight men who consumed 1,200 calories a day. Ten minutes before each meal all dieters took 3 grams of glucomannan in capsule form.

After 12 weeks the dieters had lost an average of 15 pounds. That is more than double the average 7 pounds weight loss produced on similar diets without taking glucomannan capsules the study showed.

Reading Labels For A Successful Diet For a successful diet you should read product labels. Labels must list ingredients based on the quantity of each ingredient in descending order. If sugar is the first ingredient listed, that means there is more sugar in the product than any other ingredient. Products high in sugar and salt could hamper your diet efforts.

• Labels can call sugar something else. For example, sugar can also be called sucrose, glucose, dextrose, fructose, corn syrups, corn sweeteners and invert sugar.

• Labels may call salt something else. Names such as sodium benzoate, disodium phosphate and sodium propionate are actually names for salt.

Avoid Diet Drinks--May Cause Weight Gain

Artificial sweeteners put in diet drinks can make you gain weight, says Dr. Dennis Remington, Director of Eating Disorder clinic at Brigham-Young University. Here's why:

• Artificial sweeteners are many times sweeter than sugar so they cause a craving for sweets.

• To satisfy this craving for sweets, the person is more likely to eat candy or other sugary snacks.

• The sweetness of the diet drink actually fools your system into thinking your body has ingested sugar. As a result your body releases extra insulin that can lead to weight gain.

Reducing Desire For Sweets A study published in Federation Proceedings showed that zinc can improve the ability to taste. Women showed a significant increase in the ability to taste sweetness. Getting adequate zinc in your diet may be one way to cut back your intake of sugar--and take in fewer calories.

Self-diagnosis can be dangerous. If you have a serious health problem, see your doctor promptly.

Satisfying Cravings For Snacks Snacking is one of the greatest enemies of a dieter. You must substitute low-calorie, nutritious foods for high-calorie, junk foods for a successful diet. Be prepared to have nutritious, low-calorie foods ready. The following foods are good to snack on while dieting:

- Fresh fruit such as apples, bananas, blue berries, cherries, grapes, peaches, plums and strawberries.
- Rye crackers, soda crackers with low-fat cheese, skinned chicken or turkey.
- Popcorn without butter.
- Low-fat vanilla yogurt.
- Peanuts in the shell.
- Dry, unsweetened cereal.
- Peanut butter and celery.
- Smoothies (banana or one-half cup of strawberries blended with one-cup of non-fat milk).
- Cookies with reduced sugar and whole-wheat flour.
- Bran muffins.
- Artificially-sweetened geletin.
- Raw vegetables such as cauliflower, cherry tomatoes, cucumbers, mushrooms and carrot sticks.

Other Suggestions
- Brush teeth and tongue after meals. This will discourage snacking.
- Fill up on water when you start to feel hungry.

DIGESTION

Two Common Foods That Aid Digestion Drinking one ounce of pineapple juice mixed with one ounce papaya juice with each meal is a great way to aid digestion, according to Dr. L. L. Schneider. Papaya contains the enzyme papain and pineapple the enzyme bromelain. Both enzymes promote digestion and combat excess stomach acid.

Papaya Tablets Many persons report that papaya tablets taken alone aid digestion. Even the U.S. Department of Agriculture has praised the digestive aid value of papaya. Papaya talbets are available at health food stores.

DOG BITES

How To Prevent When you're confronted with a hostile dog there are several precautions you should take to avoid being bitten.

- Never run, even if the dog rushes at you. This brings out the "chase instinct" in the dog.
- Don't show fear. It makes the dog think you are vulnerable.
- Never look a dog or any other threatening animal directly in the eye. This may lead the animal to believe he is being challenged.
- If possible, place something between you and the dog, like a package or a purse.
- Do not turn your back on the dog. Instead, turn your body sideways and back away very slowly.
- Do not try to make friends with the dog. Don't try to pet it and don't put your hands or face near it.
- If the dog does bite you, don't pull away. This will cause a tear and a worse wound.

A dog that holds its tail high and stiff and its ears up showing its teeth can be very dangerous. Conversely, a dog whose tail is down and ears back is more likely to calm down when you freeze.

DRINKING (See Also ALCOHOLISM)

Causes Loss Of Vitamins Drinking alcohol can destroy essential vitamins in your body. The three most important vitamins lost are thiamine, zinc and magnesium. Other vitamins lost through drinking are vitamin A, B-6, B-12, C, D, folic acid, riboflavin and calcium. If you drink more than 2 or 3 drinks a day consider supplementing your diet.

DRIVING

Reducing Driving Stress Driving in rush-hour traffic can be one of the most stressful things in life. Here are some tips to avoid stress while driving.

- Breathe deeply. Listen to soothing music. Think about things you need to do.
- Get comfortable. Adjust your seat so you can see 10 feet ahead. Keep your knees slightly lower than your thighs.
- Once out of the car take a short walk. Stretch your legs and cool off, says the Stress Management Center, Washington, D.C.

Driving Long Distances It's a good idea to take periodic breaks. Research shows it's good to have a snack while on break. Eating a snack seems to improve driving performance and cuts down on fatigue.

DROWSINESS

4 Tips To Help Stay Awake When you get drowsy at the wrong time and cannot get a cup of coffee or do something else to revive yourself, here are 4 tips that may help keep you awake:

- Press your knees together or press your elbows against the arms of your chair. The physical exertion will increase your blood circulation and make you more alert.

- Pinch the inside of your mouth between your teeth hard enough to jolt you out of drowsiness.
- Tickle the roof of your mouth with the tip of your tongue.
- Say something, even whispering to yourself. Speaking stimulates the brain and awakens you.

DRUG TESTING

Guarding Against Erroneous Results Many employers are now requiring urine samples to test for drug use. It is possible to test positive for marajuana use when you have not smoked marajuana. Being near other people who are smoking marajuana in a closed room or in a car can make your urine have traces of marajuana, according to an article in the Journal of the American Medical Association. People wanting to lessen the presence of drug traces in their urine can do this by drinking large amounts of water. The more water you drink, the more you dilute the urine and reduce the chances of traces of drugs showing up in a urine test.

DRY SKIN

3 Tips To Relieve
- The best way to moisturize skin is to soak in water then pat skin dry.
- Rub oil on the skin after the bath to seal in moisture.
- Avoid strong deoderant soaps. They tend to aggrevate dry skin. Use soaps containing cold cream.

EAR CARE

Keeping Ears Healthy
- Do not regularly clean your ears--they clean themselves.

• Avoid loud noises such as rock concerts and gun shots. They can permanently damage nerves and cause irreversable hearing loss. Wear ear plugs when exposed to loud noises.

Itching Ears Shampoos and hair sprays have ingredients that can make the inside of ears itch. Harsh ingredients can even irritate the ear canal.

How To Prevent Itching Ears
• When showering or shampooing your hair, plug your ears with cotton balls. Apply some vaseline to the cotton ball to create a water-proof seal.

• After swimming make sure water doesn't lodge in your ear canal. To prevent, use an eye dropper to place a few drops of baby oil in each ear canal. Let sit for about a minute. Then drain out by tilting your head to the side.

• Itching is often caused by ear wax accumulation. Never use any sharp objects (like a cotton swab or pencil) to remove it. You could push the ear wax deeper into the ear drum.

Helping Itching Caused By Ear Wax Rinse the ear canal with a rubber syringe filled with a 50/50 solution of white vinegar and water. Let the solution remain in the canal for two minutes. Then drain by tilting your head over a sink for two minutes. Repeat once every two weeks.

ECZEMA

Creams To Sooth Eczema is an inflamation of the skin marked by itching, blistering, scaling and sometimes an oozing of fluid. About a third of all visits to a skin doctor are for some form of eczema. Most experts believe eczema is caused by an allergy to substances in the enviroment. Eczema is usually worse in the winter and improves in the summer.

Apply hydrocortisone cream. If not available, any cream for irritated skin can be used. Noxema is cooling and helps reduce itching, says Dr. William Dvorine.

ELECTRIC SHOCK

What To Do If Someone Is Suffering Electric Shock
Be very careful--there is a risk of electrocution to the person trying to help. Don't touch the victim directly until the current is shut off or the person is no longer in contact with the electricity. Victims struck by lightening, of course, may be touched immediately.

Removing The Victim From The Source Of Electricity
• Turn off the current. Remove the fuse or pull the main switch if possible. If not possible call the electric company to cut off electricity.

• To remove the victim from a live wire, stand on something dry such as a newspaper, board, blanket, rubber mat or cloth. Wear dry gloves if possible. Be extremely careful.

• Push the victim away from live wire with a dry board, stick or broom handle, or pull the victim away with a dry rope looped around an arm or leg. Never use anything metalic, wet or damp. Be careful. Do not touch the victim until free from the wire.

EMOTIONS

How To Control Your Emotions
The kind of expression you put on your face helps determine how you feel inside, says Dr. Paul Ekman, Professor at the University of California, San Francisco. Research showed that by coaching students to move facial muscles a certain way their bodies also experienced like emotions of fear, anger, disgust and amusement. For example, a facial expression of fear caused the body to feel fear. Anger caused the body to feel anger. Sadness caused feelings of sadness.

Preliminary research also shows that a person can control the results of a lie-detector test by the expressions put on his face. Russians train agents to be able to control the results of lie detector tests. The Russians have done more research in this area than the U.S.

ENERGY

How To Get More Energy
• One of the best ways to get quick energy is by drinking a glass of grape juice, according to Dr. L. L. Schneider in his book "Old-Fashioned Health Remedies". Grape Juice is one of the most readily assimilated foods for quick energy.
• Taking in oxygen is another good way to get quick energy. The following walking and breathing exercise is an effective way to get more oxygen.
1. Walk at a normal pace.
2. Inhale counting as you go.
3. Exhale slowly taking twice as long as inhalation to count.
This simple exercise energizes the body by increasing oxygen levels.

EYES

Removing Minor Foreign Objects To remove a minor foreign object such as an eye lash, speck or cinder (that is floating on an eyeball or inside the eye lid) carefully follow these suggestions.
1. Do not rub the eyes.
2. Wash hands with soap and water.
3. Gently pull upper eye lid down over lower eye lid and hold for a moment. This causes tears to flow which

sometimes washes out the particle.

4. If the particle is not removed, fill eye dropper with warm water. Squeeze water over the eye to flush out particle. If eye dropper is not available hold head under gentle stream of water to flush out particle.

5. If still unsuccessful gently pull lower eye lid down. If foreign body can be seen on the inside of the lower lid, carefully lift particle out with a moistened corner of clean handkerchief, cloth or facial tissue.

6. If speck is not visible on the lower lid check the inside of upper lid. This can be done by first holding the lashes of the upper eye lid and pulling downward. You must look downward during this entire procedure. While holding the eye lid down place a match or Q-tip horizontally across the outside of the lid and flip the eye lid backward over the stick. Carefully remove particle with moistened corner of handkerchief, cloth or facial tissue. If particle still remains cover the eye with a sterile or clean compress and seek medical attention. Never attempt to remove any particle that is sticking in the eye ball. Seek medical attention for such injuries.

3 Suggestions To Avoid Eye Strain While Watching TV

- Don't have a lamp near the screen so it can cause glare.
- Stay at least 7 feet from your TV. Never sit so you have to look up at the screen.
- Be sure all lighting in the room comes from behind and does not reflect off the screen.

Avoiding Eye Strain At Work Here are some relaxation techniques that will help prevent eye strain and fatigue:

- Close your eyes for five minutes every few hours.
- Rub your hands together for a few minutes to make them warm. Lean back in a chair and cup your palms over your eyes. The heat will relax your eyes. Look out the window or down a hall. Relax and try to look as broadly as you can,

taking in everything for about 1 minute. This also tends to relax your eyes.

• Hold a pencil at arms length and pull it slowly towards your eyes until you see double. Repeat for 1 minute a day. This will help strengthen eye muscles.

FACIAL HAIR

Ways To Get Rid Of

• *Waxing.* Waxing is probably the best method for removing large areas of hair. If done correctly it can remove the root so the hair will not grow back. Be sure to buy a high quality wax that does not get brittle.

• *Shaving.* Shaving is the most popular, temporary solution to hair on the face. Of course, the hair grows back quickly. Stubble may eventually become a problem.

• *Depilatory Creams.* These creams dissolve unwanted hair leaving the skin surface smooth. But, they can create skin irritations. When using for the first time, make a patch test. Leave the product on a spot of skin for 24 hours. This will tell you whether you are allergic to the compound.

• *Electrolysis.* This is the only permanent solution to hair growth. Electrolysis destroys the hair root so it will not grow back. If done properly it is very effective. However, electrolysis can be painful and costly.

• *Bleaching.* Bleaching may be a good solution for small amounts of hair. Bleaching the hair makes it less visible. This method is preferred for certain types of hair on the face. Bleaching must be done regularly. When the hair grows back the color returns.

• *Tweezing.* Tweezing is an effective way to remove hair but it is also painful. Many people apply wrapped ice to the skin after tweezing to reduce swelling.

FALLS, PREVENTING

8 Tips For Preventing Falls Accidents seldom just happen--many can be prevented. Safety is especially important for older persons.

- Illuminate all stairways and provide light switches at both the bottom and the top.
- Provide night lights or bedside remote-control light switches.
- Be sure both sides of stairways have sturdy handrails.
- Tack down carpeting on stairs and use nonskid treads.
- Remove throw rugs that tend to slide.
- Arrange furniture and other objects so they are not obstacles.
- Use grab bars on bathroom walls and nonskid mats or strips in the bathtub.
- Keep outdoor steps and walkways in good repair.

FATIGUE

Alleviating Fatigue People visit doctors for fatigue more than any other symptom. Fatigue can be due to physical or psychological factors. Prolonged fatigue requires professional attention to determine the underlying causes.

Reducing Fatigue-Causing Conditions
- *Noises.* Noises can add to stress and trigger fatigue. Find a quiet place to work and relax.
- *Privacy.* Lack of privacy contributes to stress and fatigue. Find a place away from people.
- *Tight Clothing.* Avoid clothing that is too small or too tight. It can restrict the blood vessels and contribute to fatigue. Women should avoid tight girdles and brassiers.
- *Prescription Drugs.* Fatigue can often be caused by an

adverse reaction to prescription drugs. Ask your doctor or pharmacist about side effects of medications.

● *Sleeping Conditions.* A sagging or uncomfortable mattress can rob you of sleep and cause fatigue. Sleep on a firm, quality mattress.

● *Eye Strain.* Make sure your glasses fit well. Be sure you have the proper prescription for your glasses.

Anti-Fatigue Research For Consideration

● *Magnesium.* A deficiency of magnesium is a common cause of fatigue, says Dr. Ray C. Wunderlick of St. Petersburg, Florida. In a research study 200 men and women suffering from tiredness were given magnesium. In all but 2 cases, tiredness disappeared. This study appeared in the Second International symposium on Magnesium. Foods rich in magnesium include brown rice, bran, green vebetables, honey and sea food.

● *B Vitamins.* One of the main reasons for chronic fatigue and tiredness is lack of B-vitamins, says Dr. Lendon Smith, a nationally-known nutritional expert. A 25-milligram daily dose of B-complex is sufficient for most people to combat a deficiency. This amount of B-complex should increase energy levels and help you deal with stress better.

One reason for a deficiency is the processing that foods go through. B-vitamins are one of the first to disappear when food is over-processed. Foods rich in B-complex vitamins include brewer's yeast, wheat germ, whole grains and yogurt.

● *Potassium.* Potassium deficiency may be a cause of fatigue, especially in professional athletes and long-distance runners. This mineral helps cool muscles. Potassium is sometimes used up after hours of exertion or exercise. If it's not replaced, chronic fatigue may result. Foods rich in potassium include apricots, broccoli, lima beans, peaches, dates, figs and sea food.

● *Vitamin B-6.* A study in the International Journal of Vitamin and Mineral Research showed that elderly patients in nursing homes are often deficient in vitamin B-6. The study

80

showed that 56.6% of the patients in nursing homes were deficient in vitamin B-6. A deficiency of vitamin B-6 can cause fatigue. Foods rich in vitamin B-6 include bananas, cabbage, green leafy vegetables, whole grains and fish.

• *Wheat Germ Oil.* Wheat germ oil aids in the production of energy, says Dr. Thomas K. Cureton, Director of the Physical Fitness Institute at the University of Illinois. He has studied the effects of wheat germ oil for over 22 years. Wheat germ oil can increase energy, vitality and stamina. Wheat germ oil does not work overnight, says Dr. Cureton. It takes about 4 to 5 weeks to feel a difference. About a teaspoonful a day will do. The oil is best absorbed when taken on a relatively empty stomach after exercise. Wheat germ oil is available at most health food stores. It is also called Octacosonol.

• *Vitamin C.* Vitamin C and iron deficiencies may contribute to fatigue. Persons who receive 1,000 milligrams of vitamin C a day reported less fatigue and faster reaction times, according to a study in the Review of Czechoslovac Medicine.

Another study published in the Journal of the American Geriatrics Society surveyed 400 people about vitamin C intake and fatigue symptoms. The study showed those who took over 400 milligrams of vitamin C a day had less fatigue. Foods rich in vitamin C include citrus fruits and fruit juices, berries, cabbage, green vegetables and potatoes.

Other Factors Contributing To Fatigue
• Drinking too much coffee or alcohol.
• Boredom. Lack of specific interest or ambition.
• Stress. Your body uses energy fighting stress. Things that cause stress include money worries, family conflicts and setting unrealistic goals for yourself.
• Lack of regular exercise can also contribute to stress. Even exercising 20 minutes a day, three times a week will help reduce stress.

FEARS

Things Men Fear Most The five worst fears of men, according to Dr. William Appleton of Harvard and Dr. Harvey L. Ruben of Yale are:

- Fear of being fired. Most men base their self esteem on how well they do in their job.
- Fear of loss of health. Men fear being helpless and dependent on someone else.
- Fear of loss of physical power--especially sexual prowess.
- Fear of rejection of a loved one. Men have a fear of being abandoned.
- Fear their children will become failures. Men fear their children will be a burden on them later in life.

FEET

General Care Of Feet Most important in foot care is properly fitting shoes. Never buy shoes that need breaking in. It's normally your feet that break in, not the shoes. Shoes should have rounded toes. High heels should be avoided. Rubber heels are better--they reduce shock on your feet. Shoes should be made of rubber or canvas. The following tips will help you avoid problems:

- Wash feet daily. Rinse off all soap. Dry thoroughly, especially between toes.
- Trim nails straight across and not too short. Don't cut out or dig at corners.
- Wear clean socks. Change daily.
- Switch shoes from day to day.
- Use foot powder.

Caring For Feet--Summer Summer heat can make your feet swell up. This makes feet more susceptible to athlete's foot fungus. Foot experts recommend the following for hot weather foot care:

- Summer heat can make blood vessels dialate causing ankles to swell up. To prevent, take the weight off your feet by sitting down and raising feet off the ground. Flex your toes to get the blood pumping.
- Keep moving. Don't stand too long in one place. Standing still causes the fluids to accumulate in your feet.
- Wear comfortable shoes that are well cushioned. Make sure they are adequately ventilated.
- Dry feet thoroughly after showering. Dry very carefully between the toes and spray with an antifungal spray to keep athlete's foot fungus away.
- Bathe your feet using a two step process: Put feet in hot water for 3 minutes, then put in cold water for 1 minute. Repeat this several times. This will open and close veins and improve circulation.
- Massage feet using circular motions. This will make your whole body feel good.

Getting Shoes To Fit Right
- Buy shoes late in the day when your feet are the most swollen. If you buy them early they are likely to feel too tight a few hours later, says Dr. Barry Block.
- Make sure the largest part of your foot matches the widest part of your shoe.
- There should be a ½ inch of space between the end of your longest toe and the front of the shoe when standing up.
- Do not accept a different size than what you normally wear.
- Buy shoes made from natural, breathable material such as leather.
- The back of the shoe where the heel goes in should be stiff.
- The shoe sole should be flexible near the ball of the foot and should bend easily.

- Soles should be made of a shock absorbant material such as crepe.
- The maximum heel height for comfortable walking is 2 inches.

Preventing Odor From Shoes Smelling feet is often caused by bacteria lodged in the shoes. You can keep your shoes bacteria and odor free by following these tips:

- Always wear socks with shoes.
- Once a week air out your shoes in the sunlight. Sunlight kills germs.
- The same shoes should not be worn two consecutive days.
- Spray your shoes with an anti-bacterial spray once a week. Allow them to dry out for a day.
- Insert an ultraviolet light in your shoes periodically. This will help kill bacteria.

FINGERNAILS

Identifying Health Problems In Fingernails
- *Brittle Nails.* Brittle nails are a common problem in women. One reason may be iron deficiency. Researchers in Sheffield, England, found that nails are sensitive to iron shortages in the system. A shortage in iron can make the nails brittle. Foods rich in iron include dark green, leafy vegetables, fish, legumes and whole grains.
- *White Spots.* White spots on the nails may indicate zinc deficiency. Foods rich in zinc include sea food, spinach, mushrooms, whole grains and sun flower seeds.
- *Yellow Nails.* Yellow nails may indicate a shortage of vitamin E. They may also indicate problems in the lymph system or respiratory problems. Foods rich in vitamin E include dark green vegetables, fruits and rice.
- *White Nails.* White nails may indicate chronic anemia or liver or kidney problems.

FIREPLACE

Danger of Lead Poisoning Do not burn any colored newspapers or magazines in your fireplace. Colored newspapers contain lead. When this lead is burned it can emit dangerous levels of lead into your home. It is especially dangerous to children.

FIRES

Baking Soda For Kitchen Fires It is a good idea to keep a box of baking soda near the stove. This can be an ideal way to douse a fire. Never use water on a fire in the kitchen. This will make the fire worse in most cases.

Avoiding Kitchen Fires
• Regularly inspect appliances for frayed cords or other malfunctions.
• If an appliance gets wet or is not working properly have it serviced immediately. Do not keep using it.
• Never overload a circuit. It can overheat and cause a fire.
• When replacing a fuse always use the same size. Never use a larger fuse that could cause the circuit to overheat.
• Do not store items you often need in a place where you have to lean over the stove. When cooking do not wear clothing with loose sleeves that can catch fire on the burners.
• Keep pot handles turned-in so your children can't pull them off the stove and severely burn themselves.

FIRST AID

Suggested Items For Most Families It is a good idea to have useful medical supplies on hand for emergencies and home treatment of minor ailments.

Drug Items
- Analgesic--aspirin and/or acetaminophen. Both reduce fever and relieve pain, but only aspirin can reduce inflammation.
- Emetic--syrup of ipecac to induce vomiting and activated charcoal. Read the instructions on how to use these products.
- Antacid.
- Antiseptic solution.
- Hydrocortisone creams for skin problems.
- Calamine for poison ivy and other skin irritations.
- Petroleum jelly as a lubricant.
- Anti-diarrhetic.
- Cough syrup--non-suppressant type.
- Decongestant.
- Burn ointment.
- Anti-bacterial topical ointment.

Non-Drug Items
- Adhesive bandages of assorted sizes.
- Sterile gauze in pads and a roll.
- Absorbent cotton.
- Adhesive tape.
- Elastic bandage.
- Small, blunt-end scissors.
- Tweezers.
- Fever thermometer, including rectal type for a young child
- Hot water bottle.
- Heating pad.
- Eye cup for flushing objects out of the eye.
- Ice bag.
- Dosage spoon (common household teaspoons are rarely the correct dosage size).
- Vaporizer or humidifier.
- First aid manual.

Other Important Suggestions
- Keep all medicines out of reach of children.

- Medicines should have child resistant caps. Elderly persons who have difficulty opening such caps should ask their druggist for regular caps.
- Keep medicines in a cool, dry place away from food and other household products.
- Keep prescription and non-prescription drugs separated with clear labels.
- Check medicine chest supplies periodically. Get rid of spoiled or outdated products.
- Keep handy telephone numbers of local poison control center, physicians, hospital, rescue squad, fire and police departments. Have this list near every telephone and inside the bathroom medicine cabinet door.

FLATTENING YOUR TUMMY

The 20-Second Miracle A simple exercise to flatten your stomach takes just 20 seconds. You can do it anywhere.

- Sit upright or stand straight. Suck in your stomach holding it in for approximately 20 seconds. Then let go.
- Don't hold your breath while doing the exercise. Just breathe normally.
- Repeat the exercise several times per day. You should shoot for doing it approximately 16 times a day, says Dr. David Bachman.
- You should see results in a short time. Your abdomen will start to look flatter and feel tighter.

FLEAS

Keeping Your Pet Free Of Fleas Fleas can affect humans in addition to dogs and cats. Fleas can burrow under the skin causing inflamation and itching. Fleas may also carry diseases such as typhus and bubonic plague. (This is rare with domestic pets.) These suggestions should help rid your pet of fleas:

• At least every other day vacuum the area where your pet sleeps.
• Add brewers yeast tablets to your pet's diet. The vitamin B-1 in yeast is believed to emit an odor on skin that fleas hate.
• Wash your pet's bedding at least once a week.
• Give your pet a bath and then rinse in the following solution: Slice two lemons, including the peel, and place in a quart of boiling water for 1 hour. Let stand overnight. Strain the next morning and sponge solution onto your pet. The lemon scent repells fleas yet has a pleasant odor.

Keeping Your Home Free Of Fleas It is important to minimize the number of fleas in your home. Your pet may be free of fleas, but whenever he enters your home the fleas will jump back on your pet. A simple procedure may be effective in ridding your home of fleas. Here is what to do:

• Place a shallow dish of soapy water on your carpet over night. Place a small lamp beside it so the light shines directly onto the water.
• Fleas are attracted to light. They will jump at it, bouncing into the soapy water where they drown, according to Moira Anderson of Dog Fancy magazine.
• The soap softens the water causing the fleas to sink once they hit the water. If just plain water were used, the fleas would simply jump out of the water again.
• It is necessary to follow this method for about a week. At first, you will catch a large number of fleas. Then the number will decrease. The number of fleas caught may increase a few days later as hatched flea eggs start to be attracted to the lamp.

The rest of the room should be dark. Be sure to keep your pet out of the room so he does not disturb the bowl of water or lamp.

FLU

What To Do When Bug Strikes
• Stay in bed if possible.
• Take aspirin or acetaminophen (like Tylenol). Do not take aspirin with vitamin C. It may increase stomach irritation. (For children and teenagers, consult physician before administering aspirin).
• Avoid further complications by staying away from crowds.
• Drink plenty of liquids.
• Do not smoke. Cigarette smoking weakens resistence and lung power.
• Take vitamin C supplements. Eat properly and consult your doctor if your condition worsens.

FOOD ADDITIVES

May Be Harmful To Your Health Health experts are becoming increasingly concerned over potential harmful effects of food additives. Some food additives have been linked to allergies and other reactions.

Americans consume 5 to 10 pounds of additives in their food each year. This includes preservatives, emulsifiers, flavorings and colorings, say Texan A & M University Nutritionalists.

Here is a listing of common additives and their potential harmful effects.

• *Monosodium Glutamate (MSG).* This is a flavor enhancer. It can cause several reactions such as sleeplessness, itching, sweating, headaches and other allergic reactions.
• *Brominated Vegetable Oil (BPO).* This is added to fruit-flavored soft drinks to keep the ingredients blended. BPO can build in body fat and may cause long term effects.

89

• *Methylcellulose.* This is a thickener used in beverages, canned fruits and kosher foods. In some cases it may bring about allergies.

• *Talc.* It is used to dust chewing gum. Talc is also used as a filler in vitamin capsules. Talc may contain harmful asbestos fiber.

• *Butylated Hydrosytoluene (BHT).* This is a preservative used in many foods such as cereals and chewing gum. Studies indicate BHT may cause cancer.

FOOD POISONING

Tips For Preventing Poisoning Food poisoning can be very serious. Symptoms include nausea, vomiting, diarrhea and abdominal cramps. Medical attention should be sought if symptoms become severe or persist for more than 24 hours. About 44 million Americans suffer food poisoning each year. Here are a few tips to avoid food poisoning.

• Keep hot foods hot and cold foods cold. Hot foods should be kept at 140 degrees or greater. Cold foods need to be stored at less than 45 degrees. Food kept between these temperatures are prone to rapid bacterial growth and resulting food poisoning.

• Bacteria in raw poultry, fish and meat can contaminate cutting boards. Scrub with bleach after use.

• Do not use cans that are bulged. Avoid unusual colored food. If the food looks bad never taste for spoilage. Even a tiny amount of bacteria can cause botulism that can be fatal.

• If you become ill after eating at a restaurant, immediately notify the restaurant. The local public health department should also be notified.

Suggestions For Avoiding Picnic Food Poisoning
Food poisoning is a greater threat in the warmer months because of the difficulty in transporting food at safe

temperatures. Modern ice chests have made transportation to the picnic site easier. But there are several things you can do to minimize risk of food poisoning.

- Keep the more perishable foods at the bottom of the ice chest. Heat rises. So the bottom is colder than the top.
- Before leaving on the picnic freeze as many foods and drinks as possible. This will minimize bacterial contamination.
- Separately pack picnic items in plastic bags. If picnic includes sandwiches, keep ingredients separate until reaching picnic site.
- It's better not to transport raw chicken to picnic site. Cook at home and reheat at picnic site. Be sure cooked chicken is kept at below 45 degrees in transit.
- Ground meat is more perishable than solid pieces of meat and should be cooked first.
- Certain picnic foods are particularly prone to contamination. These include potato salad, egg and tuna salad. Be sure to keep them below 45 degrees.

Common Types Of Bacteria Causing Food Poisoning

- *Salmonella.* Common in raw meat, poultry, milk and eggs. Flies, other insects and pets can carry this bacteria. There are 1,700 types of salmonella bacteria. It is the leading cause of food poisoning deaths in America. Symptoms develop within 8 to 72 hours of eating contaminated food. Symptoms may include diarrhea, cramps, nausea and vomiting.
- *Staphylococci.* The most common bacteria causing food poisoning. Develops in meat, poultry, egg products, custards, cream-filled pastries, potato salad and many other foods. Most often caused by leaving food stand too long at room temperature. Symptoms develop within 1 to 8 hours after eating contaminated food. Symptoms include vomiting, cramps and diarrhea.
- *Escherichia Coli.* This bacteria is the main cause of traveler's diarrhea. It is often transported in the water supply

because of sewage contamination. Symptoms occur within 8 to 44 hours after ingestion and include mild to severe diarrhea.

Free Food Handling Information The federal government's U.S. Department of Agriculture maintains a toll-free telephone number where you can call to get answers to questions on handling meat and poultry. You can get quick answers on matters like how to tell if poultry and meat are fresh, how long to keep poultry and meat in the refrigerator and the freezer, how to safely care for food on picnics. The toll-free hotline number is 1-800-535-4555 (in Washington, D.C. call 447-3333).

FRECKLES

Sugar And Freckles Eliminating refined sugar from your diet may keep freckles under control. The more refined sugar in your diet, the more you're likely to have dark freckels, according to William Dufty, author of "Sugar Blues."

FROST BITE

Damages Your Skin Frost bite is damaging to the skin due to over-exposure to cold weather. Frost bite usually affects parts of the body having the poorest circulation like the ears, hands, feet and face. People with impaired circulation or diabetes are particularly prone to frost bite.

Symptoms Of Frost Bite
1. Skin appears red in the early stages. Pain is common.
2. As the frost bite develops, skin becomes grayish and appears waxy.

3. Ears feel cold and numb.
4. Pain disappears.
5. The skin may blister.

What To Do

1. Do not rub ears with snow or anything else.
2. Bring victim inside promptly.
3. Gently wrap ears in warm material.
4. Do not use heat lamps, water bottles or heating pads.
5. Do not allow victim to place frost bitten ears near a hot stove or radiator.
6. Do not break blisters.
7. Seek medical attention promptly.

Avoiding Frost Bite

• Wear footwear that is waterproof. Wear absorbent socks to help control perspiration.

• Be sure socks are the right size with ample room for toes. Socks should not restrict circulation. Avoid factors that contribute to frost bite such as fatigue, alcohol use and smoking.

• Keep feet dry and warm. It is not cold alone that causes frost bite. Dampness also causes it. If feet get damp or wet, change to warm, dry footwear at once.

• In very cold climates, supplementing the diet with about 425 milligrams a day of vitamin C may help prevent frost bite. Vitamin C helps maintain skin temperature. Foods rich in vitamin C include citrus fruits and fruit juices, berries, cabbage, green vegetables and potaotes.

GALL STONES

Persons At Risk Of Gallstones Gall stones are hardened, stone-like masses mostly formed by cholesterol.

They form in the gall baldder area and cause inflamation and discomfort. Frequently, the pain develops suddenly after meals. With strong symptoms surgery is usually warrented. A medication is now available that can dissolve the stones in some cases. Twice as many women as men develop gall stones. The following persons have an increased risk of gallstones:

- Overweight persons who frequently lose weight then gain it back.
- Women having 2 or more children.
- Those eating a high fat diet and having high cholesterol blood levels.

Avoiding Gall Stones--Preliminary Research

- *Fasting.* Long intervals between meals might increase the risk of gall stones, according to a study published in a British medical journal. The length of time between dinner and breakfast is especially crucial. Those skipping breakfast or drinking only coffee are reported to be at greater risk of gall stones.
- *Bran.* Adding bran to the diet may help provide some protection from gall stones, says Dr. D. E. W. Pomare. According to a research study, those adding bran to their diet every day significantly reduced cholesterol saturation in the bile. Cholesterol is the chief constituant of most gall stones. Dr. Pomare recommends complete unprocessed bran. The larger size of unprocessed bran is believed more effective than the smaller particles.
- *Lecithin.* According to a study published in the American Journal of Gastroenterology, 8 patients suffering gall stones were given lecithin. Lecithin reduced pain and altered bile chemistry in a way that would help dissolve the gall stones. Lecithin is available in most health food stores. Granules are much more potent than capsules. A typical lecithin capsule is 1200 milligrams. But one tablespoon of lecithin equals 10

typical capsules. Many people sprinkle lecithin granules on their cereal in the morning.

GARBAGE CANS

How To Clean Garbage cans can be a source of bacteria and disease. They should be cleaned regularly. Wash garbage pails with a borax solution. Then sprinkle some dry borax on the bottom of the pail.

GENERIC DRUGS

How To Save On Prescriptions A generic drug is an exact copy of a brand name drug. When a new drug is first developed, it is usually patented and sold under a single brand name. Drug patents run for 17 years. After the 17-year patent expires (or if there is no patent) other firms may also sell the drug under it's generic name or another brand name.

Every drug has a generic name. For example, tetracycline is the generic name for a widely used antibiotic. A physician may write a prescription for the generic name or several brand names such as achromycin or sumycin. Brand name drug products usually cost much more than generics.

Generics Just As Good Generics are just as good as brand name products. Both brand name drugs and generic versions must meet the same standards of quality set by the U.S. Food and Drug Administration. About 90 percent of all generic drugs are made by major drug firms.

Request Generics and Save If you're taking one of the following 14 most often prescribed drugs, it may save you money to ask your doctor to write a generic prescription instead.

Generic Name	Commonly Prescribed Brand Names	Purpose of Drug
Ampicillin	Amcill Omnipen Polycillin Principen	To fight infection (antibiotic)
Tetracycline	Achromycin V Panmycin Sumycin Tetracyn	To fight infection (antibiotic)
Acetaminophen/codeine	Tylenol with Codeine	To relieve pain, fever and cough
Hydrochlorothiazide	Esidrix HydroDIURIL Oretic	For hypertension and edema (diuretic)
Penicillin V-K	Pen-Vee K V-Cillin K Veetids	To fight infection (antibiotic)
Chlordiazepoxide hydrochloride	Librium	To relieve anxiety and tension
Propoxphene hydrochloride, aspirin, phenacetin and caffeine	Darvon Compound-65	To relieve pain (analgesic)
Erythromycin stearate	Erythrocin Stearate	To fight infection (antibiotic)
Amitriptyline hydrochloride	Elavil Endep	To relieve symptoms of depression
Diphenhydramine hydrochloride	Benadryl	Antihistamine (also for motion sickness and parkinsonism
Diphenoxylate hydrochloride with atropine sulfate	Lomotil	To help control diarrhea

Generic Name	Commonly Prescribed Brand Names	Purpose of Drug
Meclizine hydrochloride	Antivert	To control nausea and vomiting, and dizziness from motion sickness
Chlorothiazide	Diuril	For hypertension and edema (diuretic)
Erythromycin ethyl succinate	E.E.S.	To fight infection (antibiotic)

GOUT

Cherries May Help Gout is a form of arthritis that is believed to be inherited. It's caused by faulty metabolism of protein which causes high levels of uric acid in the system. The uric acid forms crystals which lodge in the joints--mostly the big toe. This causes considerable pain. Typical victims are men in their 40's. Women rarely suffer gout.

Some gout sufferers have reported cherries relieve the pain of gout. They say that cherries--either canned, fresh or frozen and even cherry juice concentrate--eased the pain of gout.

GRAY HAIR

One Doctor's Way To Prevent Gray Hair According to Dr. Abram Hoffer, a psychiatrist from Canada, taking an 800 IU capsule of vitamin E every day prevented his hair from going gray. The doctor brags of a healthy head of hair that is all black with no gray whatsoever. Dr. Hoffer believes gray hair is a symptom of body degeneration and vitamin E helps halt this condition. Foods rich in vitamin E include dark green vegetables, fruits and rice.

GUM DISEASE

Preventing Gum Disease About 75% of men and women over the age of 35 suffer from some periodontal (gum) disease, says the American Dental Association. For people over 60 years old, almost 40% have lost teeth because of it. Gum disease starts when plaque forms on the teeth. Plaque is a sticky film of food and bacteria that accumulates between the teeth along the gum line. If you don't remove the plaque every day it will attack your gums. With the first stages of gum disease, you gums become inflamed, may bleed and pull away from the teeth. With the second stage (Pyorrhea) of the disease, pus may ooze out of the gums. Pain may be extreme. Teeth eventually become loose and fall out. Gum disease is reversable if treated before it reaches advanced stages. The following tips may help avoid gum disease:

• *Flossing.* Careful brushing and flossing at least two or three times a day is the best defense.

• *Cleaning.* It is important to have your teeth cleaned regularly by a professional. They can get to many areas where brushing and flossing cannot.

• *Vitamin C.* Preliminary research shows that vitamin C may help protect the gums against infection. A study published in the International Journal of Vitamin and Nutritional Research showed that volunteers given 70 milligrams of vitamin C a day for six weeks showed an improvement in gum disease.

• *Calcium.* Research has shown that calcium is also a key factor in the prevention and treatment of gum disease. A calcium deficiency can weaken the bones which house the teeth and make the body more susceptable to infections, says Dr. Paul Keyes of the International Dental Foundation. Foods rich in calcium include low-fat milk, green leafy vegetables, legumes, salmon and low-fat yogurt.

Home Prevention Method Wet toothbrush in hydrogen peroxide or water. Dip the brush in baking soda and salt. Smear this mixture along the gum line. Make sure all crevices between the gums and teeth are covered, then rinse thoroughly. This method kills the bacteria and foams it away, thus helping to prevent gum disease, according to the International Dental Foundation.

Get Second Opinion A national magazine reported that many dentists specializing in gum disease (Periodontist) may prescribe unnecessary, often painful gum treatments. Reporters visited 8 periodontists in locations across the United States. One half of the periodontists visited prescribed unnecessary gum treatment. Get a second opinion.

HAIR ANALYSIS

Unreliable Results Many commercial laboratories analyze hair samples and report mineral content. This information is supposedly useful in determining what type of mineral supplements a person should take. However, a report in the Journal of the American Medical Association says that it is not possible to correlate most hair mineral levels with your nutritional status. For example, hair levels of zinc may be normal or even high in people with a severe zinc deficiency. The article says that hair analysis is only useful in cases of suspected poisoning for substances like arsenic where the presence of massive amounts of the poison in the hair would be important in making a diagnosis of the problem.

The article reports on sending 52 hair samples from 2 healthy people to 13 laboratories. The reports from these laboratories varied considerably for identicle samples. Different results for the same hair were returned from the same laboratory. Some reports from these laboratories concluded that the individual needed mineral supplements. Some laboratories offered to sell supplements to the report recipients.

HAIR CARE

11 Hair Care Tips
- Keep brushes and combs clean--they can irritate the scalp and inhibit hair growth.
- A scarf or hat will protect your hair from the sun and wind. Wear a cap to protect your hair from the chlorine in a pool. Shampoo hair immediately after swimming.
- If your hair has been permed too tight use a heavy duty protein conditioner.
- Some shampoos can cause flaking and scaling on your scalp. If this happens change your shampoo.
- To avoid damaging hair when blow-drying use a lotion or styling mousse. Don't keep the dryer too close to your hair. Don't hold it in one place too long. Keep the air moving throughout the hair.
- Split ends should be removed by cutting a quarter inch off your hair.
- To combat the frizzies use a conditioner or hot oil treatment once a week.
- Hair static can be controlled with a very light hair spray, mist or water.
- Don't fight a cowlick.
- Normal hair loses between 30 and 100 hairs a day. Don't overbrush your hair. It may cause damage and contribute to hair loss.

Self-diagnosis can be dangerous. If you have a serious health problem, see your doctor promptly.

• Never brush wet hair. Hair is very fragile when wet.

Removing Gum From Hair
To remove gum or tar from hair, rub with vegetable oil. Then wash with soap and water.

HANGOVERS

All Alcohol Not The Same Hangovers are basically caused by manufacturing by-products in alcoholic beverages called congeners, according to experiments performed at Columbia University College of Pharmaceutical Sciences in New York City. Researchers had volunteers drink an alcoholic beverage that had been poured through a charcoal filter to filter out congeners. Other volunteers drank the alcohol as it came out of the bottle. Researchers assessed hangover symptoms the next day. Those who drank the alcohol filtered through charcoal had considerably less hangover symptoms.

Alcohol That Causes The Worst Hangovers Bourbon has a high amount of congeners. People who drink bourbon are more apt to have severe hangovers, reported psychologist Dr. Loring Chapman of the University of California at Davis. Other alcohol drinks that give bad hangovers are brandy, rum, rye, scotch and red wine. All contain high amounts of manufacturing by-products called congeners. Vodka and gin have the fewest congeners. They normally provide the least severe hangover.

Getting Rid Of A Hangover Sauerkraut juice mixed with tomato juice (in equal parts) is one of the best cures for hangover, according to Dr. L.L. Schneider, a practicing physician.

HEAD CONGESTION

Try Eucalyptus Leaves The vapors of eucalyptus leaves --available in most health food stores--help clear head congestion. Place a few eucalyptus leaves in a pot of boiling water for 5 minutes then turn off the heat. With a towel draped over your head breathe the vapors. Be careful not to get too close to the steam. It could scald your face.

HEADACHE

Suggestions To Prevent Headaches Headache is one of the most common reasons why people visit a doctor. Headache pain does not originate in the brain. Brain tissues can't feel pain. Headache pain arises when blood vessels, nerves and muscles are pressured or stretched. Pain may be felt in the head, eyes and sinuses. Women report twice as many headaches as men. The following suggestions may help avoid headaches:

- Eat regular meals. Many people experience headaches when dieting or skipping a meal, says Dr. Seymour Diamond, Director of the Diamond Headache Center in Chicago.
- Don't drink too much coffee or tea. Headache sufferers often experience a caffeine withdrawal headache when they skip their daily coffee. Limit your caffeine intake to two cups a day.
- Maintain a regular sleeping schedule. Migraine headaches sometimes occur on weekends or holidays because a person sleeps past normal sleeping hours.
- Refrain from alcoholic beverages or decrease your intake.
- Don't smoke. Smoking increases blood pressure and the pressure on your brain cells.
- Avoid aged cheese and chocolate. Both can cause migraine headaches.
- Keep your hands warm. Applying heat to your hands increases the flow of blood to your brain.

- Foods that contain nitrates can cause headaches. Common foods that contain nitrates include hotdogs, bacon and other cured meats.
- Avoid chinese food if it's heavily laced with MSG (monosodium glutamate). MSG can also cause light-headedness.

Getting Rid Of Simple Headache Pain
- Try getting some fresh air.
- Lie down for awhile.
- Muscle or tension headaches are often relieved by massaging neck muscles. Heat from a heating pad or a hot tub also help.
- Eat a meal. Hunger is sometimes overlooked as a headache cause.
- Take two aspirins. Drink a cup of coffee.

Migraine Headaches This is the most common type of headache. It occurs when blood vessels in the head enlarge and press against nerves causing pain.

How To Get Relief Soaking your hands in hot water can relieve a migraine headache, say headache experts.

- When you feel a migraine headache coming on fill your sink with water as hot as you can stand it.
- Place both hands in the hot water up to your wrists for 30 minutes.
- The heat of the water expands blood vessels in your hands causing more blood to flow there. This draws blood away from bloated arteries in the head which caused the migraine headache pain.
- The hot water also stimulates nerve endings in your hands which send relaxation signals to your brain.
- The hot water takes concentration away from your pain and directs it elsewhere.

Massaging Away A Migraine Many people use a simple remedy to relieve migraine headache pain, says Dr. L. L.

103

Schneider. To relieve migraine headache take the thumb of one hand and press the palm of another. Press as firmly as you can, massaging gently. The palm has nerve endings. Pressure on the nerve endings can relieve persistent headache.

The second joint of the thumb is another spot on the hand where nerve endings affect headache. Using the thumb and index finger on the other hand rub the joint vigorously. Use oil or hand lotion to lessen friction when massaging. Repeat the process switching thumbs. If the headache is severe, 10 minutes of vigorous massage on each thumb may be required.

Magnesium A research study conducted by Dr. Kenneth Weaver, Associate Professor of Obstetrics/Gynecology at East Tennessee State University, showed that supplementing the diet with magnesium may relieve migraine headaches. In a study involving 500 women, Dr. Weaver gave them 100 milligrams of magnesium daily. Eighty percent of the women stopped having migraine headaches or they were reduced in severity. Dr. Weaver believes that most people do not get enough magnesium in their diet. You should consult your doctor before taking magnesium.

Migraines And Allergies Migraine headaches are often caused by allergies to foods, says Dr. Ellen Grant of Charing Cross Hospital in London. The doctor researched the cause of migraine headache in 60 subjects. She found the most common foods contributing to migraine headaches were wheat, oranges, eggs, figs, tea, coffee, chocolate, milk, beef, corn, cane sugar and yeast.

Herbal Remedy A controlled clinical study showed that the herb Fever Few, when taken regularly, helped prevent migraine headaches. Fever Few capsules are sold at most health food stores. According to Dr. Dean Edell, a prominent San Diego medical doctor, migraine sufferers would have nothing to lose by trying this herb for migraine headache prevention.

HEALTH INFORMATION

Call Toll-Free For Free Information This is a little-known service provided by the Federal government. To get answers to questions on any health problem simply call 1-800-336-4797 (in Virginia call 703-522-2590). A trained specialist will be available to help you. You can get answers on the telephone or get useful information in the mail.

HEARTBURN

Avoiding Heartburn Discomfort Heartburn starts when acid digestive juices and partially digested food back up into the passageway between the mouth and stomach (called the esophagus). This irritates sensitive tissues and causes "heartburn" discomfort. Here are practical suggestions for avoiding heartburn:

• Stay away from chocolate, onions and garlic. These items can cause heartburn. Avoid mixing alcoholic beverages and food. It can produce an acid stomach causing heartburn.

• Go easy on your intake of fatty foods. They contribute to heartburn. Stay away from cream sauces, gravies and salad dressings. Use just enough to flavor your food. Stay away from butter. Trim fat from your meat. Eat slowly.

• When eating sit up straight and don't wear tight clothes. Avoid girdles and tight belts.

• After eating don't drink too much coffee. Even decaffeinated coffee can cause heartburn.

• Don't smoke after a meal.

• Don't lie down after a meal. Instead, take a short walk.

• Do not eat before bedtime.

Relieving Heartburn Discomfort

• *Stand.* Merely stand or sit up straight. This forces acid and partially digested food back into the stomach.

- **Milk.** Drinking milk after eating helps combat stomach acid and brings relief.
- **Antacids.** Nonprescription antacids available in drug stores can be helpful in severe cases.

HEART DISEASE

Kills More Than Cancer Heart disease is the number one cause of death in the U.S. The most common form of heart trouble is atherosclerosis, where the artery linings become clogged by fatty deposits, shutting off the blood flow to the heart. Eating a high fat diet increases serum cholesterol in the blood and increases the chance of clogged arteries. Other risk factors are high stress, heavy smoking and high blood pressure. Men have 3 times as many heart attacks as women. One in every 2 men over 60 die from heart disease.

Prevention--Sensible Health and Diet Habits
- Don't smoke.
- Don't become overweight.
- Exercise regularly.
- Eliminate as much stress as possible from your life.
- Cut down on intake of saturated fats.

Reducing Cholesterol in Your Diet Each one-percent drop in blood cholesterol yields a two-percent reduction in the chance of coronary heart disease, says Dr. Richard A. Carleton. Thus, a five-percent drop in cholesterol brings about a 10 percent reduction in heart disease risk. A Heart Association panel recommends the following to cut cholesterol levels from your diet:
- Cut fat intake an estimated 20 percent.
- Reduce saturated (animal) fat to less than 10 percent of your total calorie intake.
- Limit poly-unsaturated (vegetable) fat to 10 percent.
- Restrict daily cholesterol intake to 250-300 milligrams a day.

Staying Alive--Research Studies Worth Considering

Fish Oil. Studies performed in the Netherlands found that people who ate fish regularly are less likely to die of heart disease than those who do not eat fish. Researchers say one or two fish dishes a week is a good idea to prevent coronary heart disease. Experts speculate the fish oil reduces fat levels in the blood and makes blood clot more slowly.

The study showed the mortality rate for those who consumed at least 14.7 ounces of fish a week was less than half that of those who consumed no fish. The researchers said, by using special methods of statistical analysis, they were able to eliminate other risk factors like cigarette smoking and high blood pressure.

Until this study the main evidence for low heart disease deaths among fish eaters came from studies among Eskimos and Japanese. These groups ate large amounts of fish and had low death rates from heart disease. Researchers say eating fish should be part of a sensible overall diet with lower saturated fats and cholesterol. The studies were published in the New England Journal of Medicine.

Aspirin. Based on a study of 11,965 men who had suffered a heart attack, the Food and Drug Administration has concluded that taking one aspirin a day is a safe and effective way to prevent another heart attack. For those who suffered a heart attack, taking one aspirin a day can reduce the risk of death by one-fifth. One regular 325 mg. aspirin is the normal dosage. Of course, people should continue to see their doctor at regular intervals to assess their progress. Aspirin appears to lessen the chance of a blood clot that can cause a heart attack. The Food and Drug Administration stresses that aspirin therapy for prevention of heart attacks is not a substitute for other preventative measures such as quitting smoking, eating a sensible diet, losing weight and exercising regularly.

Niacin. Based on a nine-year study of 8,300 male heart attack victims, niacin was found to be effective in fighting cholesterol, according to the National Institutes of Health.

The death rate of the heart attack victims taking niacin was about 11% lower than those not taking niacin daily. Niacin may be able to cut the rate of heart disease by 20-30%, according to Dr. Simeon Margolis, Professor of Medicine and Biological Chemistry at Johns-Hopkins School of Medicine. Niacin is available in most drug stores and health food stores.

Vitamin C. A British study found that male heart patients who took one gram of vitamin C daily showed a reduction in cholesterol. Cholesterol contributes to clogging of the arteries. Supplementing the diet with vitamin C can decrease the risk of atherosclerosis, says Dr. Brain Libesley, who conducted the study.

Dr. Libesley gave 25 patients one gram of vitamin C daily for 6 weeks. At the end of the 6-week period, all heart patients showed a decrease in cholesterol. Total cholesterol fell 12.5%. Foods rich in vitamin C include citrus fruits and fruit juices, berries, cabbage, green vegetables and potatoes.

Lecithin. A natural substance found in soybeans has been reported to lower cholesterol and other fats in the blood. Dr. Lester Morrison from Los Angeles, California gave 2 tablespoons of lecithin, 3 times a day (a total of 36 grams per day) to 15 people. After 3 months 12 of the 15 people showed a significant reduction in blood cholesterol. Other studies have supported Dr. Morrison's findings.

Alcohol. Drinking alcoholic beverages in moderation may protect against heart disease, according to Stamford University researchers. A study of 24 men indicated that two drinks a day lessens the risk of atherosclerosis--a narrowing and clogging of the arteries. Heavy drinking, however, can increase the chance of heart attack making you more prone to irregular and rapid heartbeat, according to the American Heart Association. Another study, supporting the benefits of moderate alcohol intake, was published in the Journal of the American Medical Association.

Beans. Preliminary studies show that beans may reduce cholesterol. A 15-month study of 242 people at Sichuan

Medical College found that cholesterol levels were lowered after adding beans to the diet for 1 to 3 months. Researchers say any kind of beans can be used, including lima beans and kidney beans. Researchers believe that beans inhibit absorption of cholesterol into the body.

Garlic. Research shows garlic may help keep the heart healthy. A study published in the medical journal Lancet examined the diet habits of 7 countries. Countries that consumed large amounts of garlic like Greece and Italy had fewer heart disease problems than other countries consuming less garlic. People who can't stand the smell of garlic can take garlic capsules, available at health food stores. The capsules are odorless and will not affect smell of breath.

Stress. You can reduce your risk of heart attack by learning how to handle stress, researchers have found. People who are hostile, aggressive and impatient--commonly referred to as type A behavior--have the greatest risk of heart attack, say researchers.

Pectin. Preliminary research indicates that pectin found in apples may help lower cholesterol levels in the blood. Many health food stores sell pectin tablets.

HEMORRHOIDS

Suggestions For Hemorrhoid Relief Hemorrhoids are swollen veins in the anus and anal area. Hemorrhoids in the anus are called external. Anal hemorrhoids are called internal. About 35 percent of the population suffers from hemorrhoids.

Hemorrhoids cause itching, burning and sometimes bleeding. Flareups can be due to habitual postponement of bowel movement, constipation and straining. Diet plays a major role in hemorrhoids. A diet high in refined foods such as white flour and sugar increases chances of hemorrhoids. The following suggestions may help avoid hemorrhoids:

- Eat bulky foods such as grains, leafy vegetables and fruits. This should help regulate bowel movements.
- Try warm water soaks to ease discomfort.
- After bowel movements, pat yourself clean with damp cloth. Avoid excess wiping with tissue paper.
- Drink plenty of liquids every day.
- Avoid lifting heavy objects.
- Use a stool softener if stool is excessively hard. Use a laxative if constipated to avoid straining (stool softeners and laxatives are available at drug stores).
- Never postpone a bowel movement. When nature calls, answer as soon as possible.

HIATUS HERNIA (DIAPHRAGMATIC HERNIA)

7 Tips For Getting Relief This condition occurs when a portion of the stomach protrudes above the diaphragm--the muscular wall separating the chest and abdominal cavity. This results in a loss of function of the valve at the bottom of the esophagus allowing stomach acid to back up into the esophagus producing heartburn--usually in the area underneath the breast bone. The pain most often occurs at night when in a reclined position. This condition may interrupt sleep. Experts estimate that about 50 percent of the U.S. population suffers a hiatus hernia. Follow this advice for relief:

- Avoid foods such as coffee, citrus fruit, highly spiced or seasoned foods and chocolate.
- Avoid eating or drinking for several hours before going to bed.
- Avoid tight fitting clothing around the waist.
- Bending should be done with the knees, not the waist, to avoid abdominal pressure.

110

- Avoid obesity, especially a pot belly.
- Elevate the head of the bed 6 to 8 inches by placing blocks under the front legs of the bed.
- Over-the-counter antacids may neutralize stomach acid and relieve heartburn.

Recent research suggests that lack of fiber in the diet may contribute to flareups. What's more, hiatus hernias are unknown in Africa. Africans eat a strict, high-fiber diet.

Studies also show those suffering a hiatus hernia are also more prone to gall stones. The reason is not known.

HICCUPS

Home Remedies To Try Hiccups are a spasm of the diaphragm. The noise is due to air being sucked in and suddenly stopped by tightened vocal cords. Millions of people suffer from hiccups every day.

Several things cause hiccups. This includes indigestion, nervousness, exercising too soon after a meal and faulty swallowing of food. Most attacks of hiccups last for less than an hour. Try these remedies for relief:

- Take a deep breath, hold it and blow out slowly.
- Drink a glass of water.
- Apply mild pressure on the eyeballs.
- Swallow a small piece of crushed ice.
- Place an ice bag on the diaphragm just below the rib cage for several minutes.
- Drink a tablespoon of lemon juice.
- Breathe and rebreathe into a paper bag.
- Swallow a teaspoon of honey or vinegar.

Massaging Roof Of Mouth Technique Massaging the roof of your mouth is the best way to stop hiccups, according to Dr. Stapczynski of the University of California, Los

Angeles. Here's how it works: Carefully place a swab in your mouth and gently massage the back area of the roof of your mouth where it is soft and fleshy for approximately one minute. This technique is effective in a high percentage of cases, according to a recent report in the Journal of the American Medical Association.

Charcoal Tablets A study published in the British Medical Journal showed that activated charcoal tablets relieved hiccups.

Participants in the study chewed charcoal tablets hourly until relief was obtained. Charcoal tablets and capsules are available at most health food stores.

HOLISTIC DOCTOR REFERRAL

Toll-Free Hotline Many people prefer going to an holistic doctor. Holistic doctors tend to view the body as one entire system as opposed to conventional medical doctors who specialize in specific areas of the body such as the eyes, the feet and intestinal tract. Holistic doctors tend to be more oriented toward nutrition and natural remedies rather than drugs and surgery. For a referral to an holistic doctor in your area call this toll-free number: 1-800-227-4458.

HUMIDIFIER

May Harbor Bacteria Humidifier units should be washed at least once a week. Scrub thoroughly with hydrogen peroxide. This will kill the bacteria and fungi that can cause respiratory problems.

HYPOTHERMIA (CHILLING OF THE ENTIRE BODY)

Ways To Help The Victim
1. Bring victim into a warm room as soon as possible.
2. Remove wet clothing.
3. Wrap victim in warm blanket, towels or additional clothing.
4. Seek medical attention promptly.

IMPOTENCE

May Be Caused By Vitamin Deficiency Impotence is most often caused by psychological factors. In only 10% of the cases the cause is physical. Impotency may also be a side effect of prescription medications. Deficiencies in zinc and vitamins A and C also may bring about impotence. Despite popular belief, vitamin E has no effect on this condition.

Sarsaparilla tea has been used by Indians in Mexico as a sexual stimulant for centuries. This tea is available in most health food stores.

Impotence Hotline To get information on impotence call toll-free 1-800-328-3863. A specialist will be available to answer your questions and send information.

Impotents Anonymous Offers help to impotent men and their partners. Many local chapters throughout the U.S. For further information write:

Impotents Anonymous
National Headquarters
5119 Bradley Blvd.
Chevy Chase, MD 20815

113

INDIGESTION (SIMPLE)

8 Suggestions For Avoiding Indigestion Simple indigestion is normally brought about by overeating, eating too fast, not chewing food properly, eating spicy or fatty foods or foods that cause an allergic reaction. Indigestion is often due to psychological factors like worry, frustration and emotional upset. Simple indigestion causes an uncomfortable feeling of fullness and slight pain in the stomach. If symptoms linger a doctor should be consulted for diagnosis. The following suggestions should help avoid problems.

- Eat meals at a leisurely pace. Don't gobble food or eat at stand up counters.
- Don't water-log food. Drink liquids before or after meals --not during.
- Eat meals in a comfortable, relaxing atmosphere. Don't discuss problems or conflicts while eating. Wait at least one hour.
- Avoid smoking before, during and after meals. Don't wear tight clothes around your midsection.
- Eat meals at regular intervals. This helps the stomach secrete digestive juices.
- Avoid large, heavy meals, especially those spicy and high in fat.
- Drink a glass of milk between meals. This will help avoid excess stomach acid.
- Avoid candy and gum. They may stimulate stomach acid.

Relieving Discomfort

- *Indigestion.* Indigestion can be soothed by effervescents like Alka-Seltzer or Bromo-Seltzer. Effervescents work quickly to neutralize stomach acids. Your best bet for occasional indigestion, says Dr. Arnold Levy of the American Digestive Disease Society.
- *Nausea.* The best antacid is one that coats and soothes the stomach lining such as Maalox.
- *Gas and Heartburn.* That bloated feeling is best treated

by anti-gas antacids like Maalox-plus or Digel. These products help break up gas bubble. (If you require antacids constantly for symptom relief you should visit a doctor immediately).

All of the products mentioned above are available in drug stores and supermarkets.

Natural Remedies For Indigestion
• *Fennel.* Fennel is an old-fashioned remedy for indigestion. Fennel is recommended in the book "Back to Eden" as a remedy for gas and acid stomach. This herb can be sprinkled on food to prevent stomach gas.

• *Anise.* The book "Nature's Healing Agents" recommends anise for a sour stomach. The anise seeds can be chewed or ground and the seeds can be sprinkled on food.

• *Mint.* Both peppermint and spearmint have been used for years as a remedy for indigestion. A cup of peppermint tea is a good remedy. It will soothe the stomach.

All of these natural ingredients are available at health food stores and most grocery markets.

Breathing Exercise To combat symptioms of stomach acid try this abdominal breathing exercise, says Dr. Nels Olson, from the University of Michigan: push out stomach with each breath rather than expanding chest.

Activated Charcoal For Stomach Gas Activated charcoal capsules, available at most health food stores, can relieve stomach gas. (Also good for diarrhea and hiccups.) Charcoal absorbs gas like a sponge. It can also absorb intestinal bacteria that can cause gas. Many people prefer charcoal capsules to any other product for stomach discomfort. If you haven't tried charcoal capsules you are missing out on one of the best stomach aids available.

Indigestion And Soapy Film Soapy film on dishes and silverware can cause problems in your digestive system. Detergent film can build up in your system and cause problems over a period of years.

Avoid Detergent Irritants
- Use a minimum of soap when washing dishes.
- Rinse everything thoroughly after washing. Be especially careful with items such as forks where residue can lodge in small areas.
- Rerinse any silverware that has a soapy taste.

INGROWN TOENAILS

4 Tips For Home Care This is the growth of a toenail into the soft tissue of the toe. It is most often caused by improperly fitting shoes. Another common cause is improper cutting of the toenails. Most people cut toenails to fit the contour of the toe. This can cause trouble. The toenail should be cut straight across without any curves. Do the following for relief:

- Soak the toe in warm salt water. Remove the dead, granulated tissue with scissors.
- Wear a cut-out-toe shoe.
- Paint the ingrown part of the nail with a 1% solution of gentian violet, available at your drug store.
- Slip a piece of cotton soaked in castor oil under the edge of the ingrown toenail to keep it pointing upward and out.

INSECT BITE

4 Tips For Avoiding Insect Bites Many people experience severe allergic reactions to insect bites. These reactions could include dizziness, nausea, diarrhea, itching and difficulty breathing. If you have a serious reaction to an insect bite see a doctor immediately. Follow these rules to avoid problems:

• When you're outdoors cooking or eating be careful. Food and drink often attract insects.

• Don't wear open shoes or loose fitting clothes. Avoid bright colored clothing that may attract insects.

• Don't use perfume or hair spray lotions or any other cosmetics. They, too, may attract insects.

• Be careful when gardening, Wear a hat and long sleeved shirt, boots and gloves.

What To Do When Bitten

• Scrape out any stingers with your fingernail or a dull knife. Do not try to pull a stinger out. Squeezing will only inject more venom into the wound.

• Wash the bite with soap and water. Then apply antiseptic.

• Apply an ice pack and/or a paste of baking soda and water to relieve pain.

• Elevate the arm or leg to reduce fluid retention and swelling.

Using Your Anti-Perspirant The active ingredient in anti-perspirants sold in drug stores is aluminum chloride. This ingredient relieves itching, pain and inflamation from insect bites, says Dr. Walter Shelley of the Medical College of Ohio. The aluminum chloride dries the skin and kills the bacteria to prevent infection. The anti-perspirant should be applied to insect bites about once every 10 hours.

IRON

Women Need More The monthly blood loss during menstruation may cause an iron deficiency in women, according to an article in the Federal government's FDA Consumer. A loss of 15 to 20 milligrams of iron occurs during a typical menstrual period. About 10 percent of all women may need twice that much, including many wearing IUD's.

Fatigue A Common Symptom Iron deficiency can cause fatigue, headache and pale complexion. Increasing evidence indicates that even a mild depletion of iron reserves may impair mental and physical performance.

Daily Iron Need The National Research Council recommends that women consume 18 milligrams of iron daily. The body only absorbs about 10 percent of the iron in food.
• Vitamin C helps absorption. Dr. James Cook, Professor of Medicine at the University of Kansas Medical Center, found that taking 66 milligrams of vitamin C with meals can increase absorption of iron up to 500 percent.
• Drinking tea interferes with iron absorption because it contains tannic acid and phytates. Antacids also diminish iron absorption.

ITCHING

2 Suggestions For Relieving Itching Skin
• According to an article in the Journal of the American Medical Association, 60 milligrams of iron, taken 3 times a day relieved itching in persons who suffered severe itching.
• A 20-minute, lukewarm bath with bath oil added is very good for dry, itching skin, says Dr. B. Allen Flaxman. The warm water tends to open pores allowing the oil into the skin bringing comfort and relief from itching.

JET LAG

Anti-Jet Lag Diet The Anti-Jet Lag diet is helping countless numbers of travelers quickly adjust their body's internal clocks to new time zones. It is also being used by persons working swing shifts who have to periodically rotate their working hours. The diet was developed by Dr. Charles F. Ehret of Argonne Division of Biological and Medical Research.

How To Avoid Jet Lag

1. Determine breakfast time at destination on day of arrival.

2. Start your Anti-Jet Lag diet three days before your departure date. On day one "feast". Eat heartily with a high-protein breakfast and lunch and a high-carbohydrate dinner. Drink no coffee except between 3 and 5 p.m. On day two, fast on light meals of salads, light soups, fruits and juices. Again, no coffee except between 3 and 5 p.m. On day three "feast" again. On day four, departure day, fast. If you drink caffeineated beverages have them in the morning when traveling west, or between 6 and 11 p.m. when traveling east.

3. Break your final fast at breakfast time at your destination. Have no alcohol on the plane. If your flight is long enough sleep until normal breakfast time at your destination, but no later. Wake up and feast on a high-protein breakfast. Stay awake and active. Continue your meals according to meal times at your destination.

JOB BOREDOM

Overcoming Boredom

• Change the way you go to work. If you drive your car, take a different route--a more scenic one. If you go to work using public transportation consider joining a car-pool.

• When at work do the most difficult tasks first.

• Move your desk or sit at a different location.

• Seek new assignments and new responsibility.

• Volunteer for activities outside of work such as baseball or football teams.

• Change your work habits. Go someplace different for lunch or try eating lunch with new employees.

JOCK ITCH

3 Suggestions For Relief Jock itch is a fungus infection around the genital area. It strikes males who regularly engage in vigorous exercise. Moisture and friction cause the fungus to grow.

- Quickly change sweaty and soiled clothing.
- Wear jockey type shorts instead of the baggier boxer shorts.
- Sprinkle affected area with Tinactin powder after bathing.

JOINT INJURIES

Home Remedies For Minor Problems
- *Rest.* Stop using the injured joint as soon as you feel pain, says Dr. Charles Bull.
- *Ice.* Place a towel over the injured joint and apply an ice pack over the towel.
- *Compression.* Wrap an elastic bandage over the ice and around the injured part to limit swelling. Leave the ice pack and bandage in place 20 minutes of wrapping and 20 minutes of unwrapping for 3 hours.
- *Elevation.* Position the injured part so that it is above the level of your heart so that gravity will help drain excess fluids.
- Continue treatment for up to 24 hours.
- Consult a doctor if your pain is severe or lasts more than one week.

KNOCKED OUT TEETH

What To Do Wrap the knocked out tooth in a cool wet cloth. Take the victim and the tooth to the dentist as soon as possible. A destist can often reimplant the tooth with a high degree of success.

LAUGHTER

May Fight Disease And Pain Laughter stimulates the brain to produce hormones that fight disease and pain, according to Dr. William Fry of Stamford Medical School in California. Laughter is like an innoculation against disease. Without laughter people get sick more often. Hormones generated by laughter reduce tension--a major cause of pain. Laughter is also good for guilt and depression.

LEG CRAMPS

Tips That May Help Leg cramps due to muscle spasms is a common problem, especially among older people. Cramps most often happen at night. The discomfort can be relieved by walking or moving the leg. Also consider these nutrients:
  • *Calcium.* Supplementing your diet with about 900 milligrams of calcium per day can ease leg cramps caused by muscle spasms, says Dr. Ralph Smiley of Dallas, Texas.
  • *Vitamin E.* Supplementing the diet with 100 I.U.'s of vitamin E with each meal may help ease leg cramps.

LICE

How To Prevent And Treat Lice are parasites that infest the body, especially hairy parts They can cause severe itching and tiny red marks on the skin. Lice are often carriers of typhus.

Self-diagnosis can be dangerous. If you have a serious health problem, see your doctor promptly.

121

How Transmitted Lice can be transmitted by personal contact, use of a borrowed comb, brush, hat or other clothing. The white lice eggs attach to the hair and mature in 3 to 14 days.

Treatment A safe insecticide in cream form or lotion available at a drug store should be applied to all hairy surfaces and rubbed into the scalp at night. In the morning shampoo thoroughly. Repeat this treatment in a week to catch any lice that have survived or have been newly born.

Tips To Prevent Periodically sterlize hats, brushes, combs and other clothing that go on the head. Thoroughly launder (or boil) bed linen and towles. Avoid all body contact until lice disappear.

LIVING LONGER

What You Can Do Now The American Longevity Association has ten tips to help you live to be 100 or over. Here are the Association's recommendations:

- Substitute fish for meat as often as possible. Fish contains oils that may prevent heart attacks. (Heart disease is the #1 cause of death in America.)
- Use fish oils and olive oil in salads and cooking. Research has shown these oils lower cholesterol.
- Substitute vegetables for meat and dairy products.
- Increase your intake of foods high in beta carotenes such as carrots, spinach, broccoli and cantaloupe. This helps prevent cancer. (Cancer is the #2 cause of death in America).
- Stay on a basic low-fat diet to prevent heart disease and cancer.
- Keep your caloric intake and weight low to help slow aging.
- To help keep body tissues healthy eat more foods high in vitamin C (citrus fruit, green vegetables, green peppers, etc.).

- Eat foods high in vitamin E (vegetable oils and grains), zinc (pork, pumpkin seeds), and selenium (bran, tuna, fish).
- Substitute hard water for soft water. Also, use a charcoal filter to help eliminate chlorine from your water and remove cancer-causing materials.
- Don't smoke.

10 Old-Fashioned Rules According to Dr. L. L. Schneider, in his book "Old Fashioned Health Remedies," the 10 rules for longer life are as follows:

1. Get 7 to 8 hours sleep each night.
2. Eat 3 well-balanced meals a day.
3. Eat bulk foods and mineral and vitamin enriched foods daily.
4. Cut down on sugary foods and chemically-treated foods.
5. Get fresh air and sunshine every day if possible.
6. Drink a few glasses of fresh water each day.
7. Do not smoke. Stay away from people who do smoke.
8. Avoid alcoholic drinks except rarely and then in moderation.
9. Exercise naturally every day. Walking, swimming or gardening are good.
10. Use laughter to banish anxiety and fear. Let everyday be joyous.

MARITAL CHEATING

About 1 In 4 Spouses Cheat Marital cheating can be bad for your health when your mate finds out about it. Researchers say that about 26% of husbands and 21% of wives have love affairs with other partners.

MEDICINES

How To Tell If Spoiled Always check expiration date. Then check for signs of deterioration as follows:

• *Solutions And Liquids.* Odor, taste and color should be same as when originally purchased.

• *Pills And Tablets.* They should retain original size, weight, color. Splits, cracks and chips are a sign of decay. Also watch out for any unusual odor.

• *Capsules.* Capsules should not be too soft. They should not stick together. They should not crack under pressure.

• *Ointments.* Consistency should be same as when originally purchased. Ointments should not be harder or softer than when originally purchased.

MEMORY

Lecithin And Memory Improvement A study conducted at the National Institute of Mental Health showed that lecithin significantly improved memory and recall in normal healthy people. After taking lecithin, volunteers were able to remember a sequence of unrelated words more quickly. This study was published in the Life Sciences Medical Journal. Lecithin is available in health food stores.

MENTAL HEALTH

Problems Can Strike Anyone One in four American families is affected by mental illness. No segment of our society is immune. Mental illness can affect anyone--rich or poor, educated or not educated. It can strike at almost any age.

The picture is not bleak, however. People do recover from mental illness. There are some famous examples including President Abraham Lincoln, novelist Virginia Wolfe, U.S. Senator Thomas Eagleton, popular singer Rosemary Clooney and professional golfer Bert Yancey. All suffered from mental illness but totally recovered.

Abraham Lincoln, for example, suffered from severe depression. Only after he overcame this affliction did he attain the Presidency and become one of the world's most outstanding leaders. Lincoln is not alone in having achieved great success despite struggles with mental illness. There are thousands of cases of men and women who have suffered from mental illness--have recovered and risen to great heights of success and happiness.

If you or someone else is affected by any type of mental illness do not get discouraged. The vast majority of people recover and go on to lead happy, productive lives. Moreover, most people during their lifetime experience difficult periods that can be considered some form of mental illness.

Warning Signals Of Mental Illness While not necessarily definate signs of mental disturbances, the following signs of trouble can sometimes help you identify someone who needs help.

• Is the person acting differently than he usually does? Can you link this change in behavior to something that has happened recently?

• Does the person seem to be excessively withdrawn and depressed? Are hobbies, friends and relatives ignored suddenly? Is there a feeling this person has begun to lose confidence? Depressive illnesses have many symptoms similar to these.

• Does the individual complain of episodes of extreme, almost uncontrolable anxiety? Is this anxiety unrelated to any normal concern such as a child's illness or a backlog of bills? Anxiety having no recognizable cause is a sign of emotional difficulty.

• Does the person become aggressive, rude and abusive over minor incidents? Are there remarks about individuals or groups out to get him? This is an indication that some help may be required.

• Is there any change in the person's habits such as eating, sleeping or grooming? Suddenly, has the individual almost stopped eating? Conversely, has the person started eating or drinking a lot in a compulsive manner? Either sleeplessness or too much sleeping can be indicators if they are done in excess.

Any of these signals, if they continue for any length of time may call for professional help.

What To Do In Emergency Situations If a person becomes violent, gets completely out of control or even tries to commit suicide, there are several things you can do.

• Call a physician. Call the person's family doctor if he has one. If not, get the person to a hospital where there are doctors on duty in an emergency room.

You may have to call an ambulance to get the person there. Look in the yellow pages under ambulances or call the police or fire department or rescue squad if any of these provide ambulance services in your community. Look under the list of emergency numbers in the front of your phone book or call the operator if you can't find the number in a hurry. The operator may be able to connect you with the service you need or give you a number to call.

Also, many clergy are trained to deal with emergencies or they can refer you to the right help.

• If the victim is already in treatment, call his therapist.

• Call the mental health hotline, drug hotline, suicide prevention center, free clinic or alcoholics anonymous chapter in your area. These telephone lines are often manned around the clock. Look for the number under emergency numbers in the front of your phone book or you can find a listing in the white pages or ask the operator for help.

• Call the nearest community mental health center. If it's not listed that way in the phone book, look for it under

126

hospitals, clinics or physicians in the yellow pages.

• In crisis emergencies call the police. Often the police are the best equipped, most available resource, especially when a crime has been committed or when there is a strong possibility that the person may do physical injury to himself or others.

Treatment Methods Here are some of the modern methods of treatment to help overcome problems.

Short-Term Psycho-Therapy This approach is used when the problem seems to be brought on by some event or episode in life such as a death in the family, divorce or physical illness. Even good news can sometimes cause a severe upset. A job promotion or a move to a better home are good examples. The goal of the therapy is to help iron out the problem as quickly as possible. Often, this takes only a few visits.

Family Therapy In this method, the whole family is interviewed to help determine the root cause of a problem. Perhaps the son needs to be with his father more. A mother may be spending too much time worrying about things that would be less of a problem if she could see them in a different way. If the family therapist can lead the family members to see each other in a new light, their behavior towards one another can improve and their problems begin to fade.

Group Therapy Group therapy takes place when a small group of people gather to discuss their common problems under the guidance of a therapist. The group members help each other with their individual problems. The therapist guides the conversation into useful directions, offers advice if needed and points out things the group members might otherwise miss.

Other Treatments There are other kinds of psycho-therapy. Some involve an in-depth study of the underlying causes of a problem that started in childhood. Other therapies deal more with the person's life here and now. Everyday situations are looked at to help the patient better understand himself.

Where To Go For Help: Paying For The Services If you are financially able to pay for psychological counseling, there are a large number of qualified professionals listed in your telephone book. You have your choice of going to a psychiatrist, who is a trained medical doctor or a psychologist.

If you believe you cannot afford psychological counseling you can start by contacting your local Community Health Center. There are more than 700 of these centers throughout the country. They are funded by the federal government and are operated by state and local agencies. The cost of the services should depend on what you can afford to pay. So if you have no money or very little, services are provided on a sliding scale. To find the Community Health Center nearest your home call your local Federal Information Center. Ask the information specialist for the number of the Community Health Center nearest your home.

The Most Common Types of Mental Problems The most common problems in today's society are anxiety and depression. Each of these problems is described below.

Anxiety Anxiety is a fearful anticipation of something. The fear may be real or imagined. Either way it feels the same. Everyone at one time or the other has experienced mild anxiety. It is only when these feelings of anxiety become severe that they cause problems. To feel anxiety is to feel fearful, scared, jittery, edgy, concerned, worried, helpless, insecure, uptight. Most of these feelings involve uncertainty over one's personal safety. The intensity of the anxiety depends on the real or imagined severity of the impending loss, the closeness of the threat and the importance of the loss to the individual.

When we experience anxiety certain hormones, especially

adrenalin, shoot through our bodies and can cause physical symptoms such as sweaty palms, rapid pulse, increase in blood pressure, dizziness and a wide variety of other physical sensations. Severe anxiety is often described as panic, where a person can feel disoriented, detached, frantic, with wierd feelings and sensations. They may think they are going crazy or will lose their mind or lose control of themselves. This can be a very disabling problem. The fear of panic can be so severe it can cause a condition referred to as agoraphobia, where the person is afraid of leaving the home for fear of having a panic attack. Anxiety and panic conditions can often be successfully treated through psycho-therapy. Complete professional treatment programs for those suffering anxiety, panic and phobias are available throughout the country. One successful program is called TERRAP. This is a 16-week program that deals with persons specifically suffering from fear, panic and anxiety. You can find out about the TERRAP program by referring to your local phone book or calling your local community Mental Health Clinic.

People suffering severe anxiety are often prescribed anti-anxiety medications such as valium, librium or xanax. These medications are highly effective in controlling anxiety during the time the person is solving the root cause of the problem through some kind of therapy.

Avoid Sugar. Three studies by the National Institute of Mental Health revealed that 75% of patients suffering from anxiety and panic disorders had a dramatic increase in anxiety after eating sugar. Moreover, 50% of people not suffering from anxiety also experience a higher level of anxiety after eating sugar. The sugar consumed during the study was equivalent to 1 to 2 slices of cake or 1 to 2 candy bars daily. Researchers suspect that sugar may cause the body to release too much of the hormone adrenalin. Adrenalin is the major culprit in causing physical reactions and panic attacks.

Caffeine. According to an article in the New England Journal of Medicine, caffeine triggers the release of adrenalin which can cause heart arrhythmia, stress and panic reactions.

Depression It is estimated that over 30 million Americans suffer some form of depression. As many as 1 in 5 of us will experience depression sometime in our lives. Women suffer depression twice as often as men. Depression, unlike occasional blue days everyone experiences, is a persistent disorder. It can bring on physical as well as mental symptoms.

Some common symptoms of depression include:
- Getting little or no pleasure out of anything in life.
- Losing interest in your job, family life, hobbies or even sex.
- Experiencing frequent and unexplained crying spells.
- Feeling a loss of self-esteem.
- Becoming unusually irritable.
- Having trouble sleeping, especially waking up at early hours and not feeling well.
- Difficulty concentrating and remembering.
- Experiencing physical pain you can't pin down.
- Loss of appetite and constipation.

Depression in most cases can be easily diagnosed and successfully treated. New effective anti-depressant drugs can shorten the course of depression. These drugs help many people to function day-to-day, keeping their jobs and relationships intact.

The most widely used anti-depressant class of drugs are called tricyclics. Experts say that about 80% of those on the right dosage of tricyclic drugs eventually get better. Some of the common tricyclic drugs are Elavil, Norpramine and Adapin. These medications are usually taken before going to bed and provide relief throughout the day. These anti-depressant drugs usually take about two weeks before they are effective in helping lift depression.

Doctors also suggest certain lifestyle changes that can help avoid and relieve depression. Among these are regularly exercising, thinking positive thoughts, maintaining social contacts as much as possible, eating a balanced diet, participating in hobbies and recreational activities and maintaining close family ties.

Sources of Further Information Excellent sources of information include:

- Mental Health Association
  800 North Kent Street
  Rosslyn, VA 22209
  telephone: 703-528-6405

- Family Service Association of America
  44 East 23rd Street
  New York, NY 10010
  telephone: 212-674-6100

If you believe you or someone you know can benefit from the services of a Community Mental Health Center or one of the facilities described above, don't delay. Please get help as soon as you can.

MICROWAVE OVEN SAFETY

Microwave Ovens And Your Health Microwave radiation can heat body tissue the same way it heats food. Exposure to high levels of microwaves can cause a painful burn. The lense of the eye is particularly sensitive to intense heat, and exposure to high levels of microwaves can cause cataracts. Likewise, the testes are very sensitive to changes in temperature. Accidental exposure to high levels of microwaves can alter or kill sperm production causing temporary sterility. Less is known about what happens to people exposed to low levels of microwaves. Research is continuing in this area.

Checking Microwave Ovens For Leakage There is little cause for concern about excess microwaves leaking from ovens unless the door hinges, latches or seals are damaged, or if the oven was made before 1971. All microwave ovens made after October 1971 are covered by radiation safety standards enforced by the Food and Drug Administration (FDA). Most ovens tested by the FDA show little or no detectable microwave leakage.

If there is some problem and you believe your oven might be leaking, contact the oven manufacturer, a microwave repair service, your state health department or the nearest FDA office. Most oven manufacturers will arrange for your oven to be checked. Many states have programs for inspecting ovens. A limited number of microwave ovens are also tested in homes by the FDA as part of its overall program to make sure that ovens meet safety standards.

Tips On Microwave Oven Operation

● Follow the manufacturer's instruction manual for recommended operating procedures and safety precautions for your own model.

● Don't operate an oven if the door does not close firmly or is bent, warped or otherwise damaged.

● Never operate an oven if you have reason to believe it will continue to operate when the door is open.

● Don't stand directly against an oven and don't allow children to do this for long periods of time while in operation.

MOLD

Source Of Harmful Bacteria Mold on fruits can be a source of harmful bacteria. It can also cause allergies. Mold on fruit goes much deeper than what appears on the fruit. It is a good idea to dispose of fruit containing any kind of mold at all.

MORNING SICKNESS

3 Suggestions To Help Avoid Morning sickness is the term used to describe the feeling of nausea that occurs in the early weeks of pregnancy. Try the following for relief:

- Eat before getting out of bed in the morning. If you cannot eat a full breakfast, tea and crackers are the next best thing.
- Instead of eating three regular meals eat several small meals.
- After eating lie down for about 20 minutes.

Vitamin B-6 Many women have reported relief by supplementing their diet with vitamin B-6. Dr. Dean Edell, a San Diego physician recommends taking no more than 75-100 mgs. a day.

Ginger Root Capsules Ginger root capsules are commonly used for motion sickness. But many women take them for relief of morning sickness, according to Dr. Dean Edell. Ginger root capsules are available at most health food stores.

Morning sickness may be a good sign. Studies show that women having morning sickness are more likely to have a healthy baby.

MOSQUITO BITES

2 Suggestions For Avoiding Bites Mosquito bites should be avoided. Mosquitos can also spread encephalitis (inflamation of the brain) and yellow fever. Try these suggestions for avoiding mosquito bites:

- *Vitamin B-1.* Researchers at Lake Superior State College in Michigan conducted a study on 60 volunteers. Thirty of the volunteers took a vitamin B-1 supplement, and the other 30 took a fake pill. Volunteers then went outdoors, keeping track of any mosquito bites. Those who took the vitamin B-1 supplement reported fewer insect bites. Your body's supply of vitamin B-1 can be depleted by excess intake of sugar and alcohol. Foods rich in vitamin B-1 include brown rice, brewer's yeast, wheat germ, blackstrap molasses and fish.

● *Refined Sugar.* Eliminating refined sugar from your diet causes mosquitos not to bite you, according to William Dufty, author of the book "Sugar Blues". Eliminate refined sugar from your diet for at least a year and mosquitos will leave you alone, says Dufty.

When refined sugar is eaten the skin lets off a sweet scent that attracts mosquitos. When sugar is eliminated the skin no longer produces this scent. Mosquitos won't bother you.

MOTION SICKNESS

Using Ginger Root To Prevent A recent study showed that 2 capsules of powdered ginger root, available at health food stores, was twice as effective in stopping motion sickness as 100 milligrams of dramamine.

Preventing Motion Sickness In Children A study published in the New England Journal of Medicine showed that elevating a child in the back seat may prevent motion sickness. When a child is sitting normally in a seat his eyes cannot focus on fast moving objects. He sees only vibrating and bobbing objects. This can cause motion sickness. When the seat is raised he can focus on relatively still objects-- reducing the effects of motion.

Other Suggestions
● Sit where there is the least motion. In a car, that would be the front seat looking straight ahead. In an airplane, select a seat over the wing. On a ship, stay in the middle section on the deck rather than below.

- Lie in a semi-reclined position and keep your head as still as possible.
- Look ahead at the horizon or close your eyes if watching passing scenery makes you ill.
- Focus on something other than the motion. For example, occupying children with coloring books may be better than having them look out the window.
- When using a product to prevent motion sickness, such as ginger root or Dramamine, take 30 minutes to an hour before traveling. These products generally do not provide relief after the onset of symptoms.

NAILS

How To Care For Them

- *Brittle Nails.* Keep fingernails well moisturized. Use nail polish remover as little as possible. Buffing nails smooths them and removes debris. Avoid contact with detergents and chemicals. Supplementing diet with iron may help. Foods rich in iron include dark green leafy vegetables, fish, legumes and whole grains.
- *Hangnails.* Cut off with sharp scissors. Proper moisturizing and wearing gloves while doing work is the best way to prevent hangnails.
- *Ingrown Toenails.* Cut toenails straight across so there are no edges to grow into the flesh. In severe cases consult your physician. (Also see section on ingrown toenails).

NASAL CONGESTION

Unclogging The Nose Nasal congestion occurs when blood vessels in the nose enlarge, taking up space in the nasal cavity. This restricts the amount of air allowed in for easy breathing.

Self-diagnosis can be dangerous. If you have a serious health problem, see your doctor promptly.

135

• **Hot Soup.** One study showed that hot soup speeds the flow of mucus out of the nose. Adding cayenne pepper and onion may hasten relief.

• **Eucalyptus.** Place eucalyptus leaves in a pot of boiling water for 5 minutes. Turn the heat off and, with a towel draped over your head, lean over the pot and breathe in the herbal vapors. Be careful not to burn yourself.

• **Nasal Decongestants.** Nasal sprays, drops and inhalers work by shrinking swollen blood vessels in the nose. Overuse tends to "tire" blood vessels in the nose, making congestion worse over time.

NECK TENSION

Simple Exercise May Help Muscles in the neck area can become tense due to stress, working in an uncomfortable position and many other reasons. Try this exercise for relief:

1. Roll your head around your shoulders. Roll first one way then the other way.
2. Pull in your chin as far and hard as you can. At the same time, stretch the back of your neck.
3. Lean your head on one side and then another. Hold the cords of your neck tightly.

Vibrator Massaging the neck with a good quality vibrator is one of the best ways to quickly relieve neck tension. Vibrate the neck muscles on each side of the vertebrae and along the top of the shoulders. The intense vibration exhausts the muscles to the point of complete relaxation. After vibrating, apply alcohol or an analgesic for a more lasting effect. Regular vibrating treatments will control neck tension.

136

NERVOUS TENSION

2 Simple Tips To Relieve Tension

Massage Hands. Massaging the web structure of the hand between the finger and thumb helps relieve nervous tension, according to Dr. L. L. Schneider in his book "Old Fashioned Health Remedies That Work Best". Apply hand cream for lubrication before starting. There are many nerve endings in the webbing between thumb and fingers. Start with the left hand. Repeat on the opposite hand for 5 minutes, twice a day or until tension is relieved.

Anti-tension Breathing Exercise

1. While standing, place both hands high on the rib cage as near the arm pits as possible.

2. Press inward as far as possible with both hands at the same time, exhaling through the open mouth.

3. Suddenly release both hands at the same time.

4. Inhale deeply holding the breath for 5 seconds. Repeat this exercise 3 to 6 times.

NIGHT BLINDNESS

Preventing Night Blindness Night blindness (nyctalopia) is a condition where a person can see well in daylight but not in fading or dim light. Night blindness is often due to a deficiency of vitamin A.

Vitamin A Supplements Night blindness can often be prevented by supplementing the diet with 2500 to 7500 I.U.'s of vitamin A a day.

Heavy Drinkers Heavy alcohol appears to interfere with the liver's ability to store and release vitamin A into the system. Heavy drinkers should consider supplementing their diet with vitamin A.

NOSEBLEED

How To Stop Nosebleed occurs when a blood vessel in the inner lining of the nose breaks. Nosebleeds are commonly due to breathing dry air for long periods, repeated blowing and injury. The following steps can help:

- While sitting up pinch your nose between your thumb and index finger. Pinch just hard enough to stop the bleeding but not enough to cause pain.
- Breathe slowly through your mouth as you continue to apply pressure for 5 minutes without interruption.
- If the bleeding doesn't stop, try again. After 3 attempts get medical help.

NOSE DROPS

Best Way To Administer Lie on your back and tilt your head backward. Put the drops in each nostril. Remain in the same position until the medication has reached your sinuses. This should take about 2 to 4 minutes.

Clean the dropper with water and wipe with tissue before placing back in the bottle. This will prevent contamination.

ODORS IN THE HOME

One Natural Way To Deoderize Home Deodorizers and sprays available in supermarkets sometimes cause allergies. Try this natural way to rid your home of odors. Douse a few cotton balls in wintergreen oil. Place these cotton balls in bathroom, kitchen and other rooms you want deodorized.

OSTEOPOROSIS

Need For More Calcium This is a condition where the bones become brittle and fracture easily due to loss of calcium. If allowed to progress the spinal column may become curved due to body weight. The victim may also lose several inches in height. Osteoporosis is the cause of the "hump back" look in so many older persons.

Medical experts agree that most women need more calcium in their diets. Some doctors are even recommending calcium supplements.

U.S. Recommended Daily Allowance (RDA) The RDA for calcium is 1,000 milligrams for adults. But experts say actual intake for adults is only 450 to 550 milligrams a day. Women who have passed menopause may need as much as 1,500 milligrams daily. Persons with a history of kidney stones should consult a doctor before using calcium supplements.

Sources Of Calcium Milk and other dairy products, fish, oranges and leafy, green vegetables are major sources of calcium. A cup of low-fat yogurt contains 350 to 450 milligrams of calcium. A cup of skim milk has 300 to 350 milligrams.

Vitamin D is needed for optimal calcium absorption. The best time for women to take calcium supplements is at night, according to Dr. Morris Notelovitz, Professor of Obstetrics and Gynecology at the University of Florida. Foods rich in vitamin D include milk, salmon, tuna and sardines.

PAIN

Cold For Relief Cold is the best remedy for the pain of injury, says Dr. H. Paul Bauer, Director of the Sports Thrapy and Body Mechanics clinic in San Diego, California. Applying ice will provide the following benefits:

- It numbs the affected area of pain.
- It decreases swelling by cutting down the blood supply.
- Experts recommend leaving the ice on for 10-15 minutes at a time. Ice is preferred over heat for treating injuries such as sprains, bruises and torn muscles.

Pain And Tryptophan Research Preliminary studies showed that l-tryptophan can help increase a person's tolerance to pain. L-tryptophan is an amino acid available in most health food stores or drug stores.

The studies involved 30 subjects who were tested on their ability to tolerate pain with a device that sends jolts of electricity to the tooth pulp.

Fifteen of the subjects took 2 grams of l-tryptophan daily for a week. The other fifteen took a fake pill. When the subjects were retested at the end of the week, the fifteen who had taken l-tryptophan were able to tolerate twice the pain as the fifteen who had not taken the amino acid. Check with your own physician before taking l-tryptophan, experts advise.

Another study published in Oral Surgery showed that patients who took l-tryptophan while undergoing root canals experienced less pain than those taking a fake pill. Patients took 2 grams of l-tryptophan spread out in 6 doses of 500 milligrams each.

PETS

Good Effects On People A number of studies have shown that pets can have a good effect on health. For example, according to a public health study, pet owners have a greater survival rate after heart attack. Other studies show that a dog can significantly lower blood pressure and reduce stress in children. Even fish and birds can have a beneficial effect on health. People tend to be more relaxed around pets. With a dog people often feel more safe.

Possible Bad Effects On People
● Numerous diseases can be transmitted by pets. One common carrier of disease is dog feces. According to a study conducted in Savannah, Georgia, a single deposit of dog feces produced an average of 144 house flies. House flies may carry disease.

● Dog bites are a nationwide problem. One person in every 250 in the United States is bitten annually.

PIMPLES

How To Stop Flareups
● When a pimple starts to become visible, apply ice for a few seconds every ½ hour. This should cause it to subside in a few hours. If it doesn't, apply a moist compress every hour.

● To take the red out of a blemish, combine one tablespoon of lemon juice with one tablespoon of salt. Apply this mixture directly to the redened area and leave it on for 10 minutes. Then rinse.

● To get rid of a pimple overnight, dip a Q-tip in witch-hazel and apply it to the pimple to dry it up. Then apply calamine lotion.

POISONING, AVOIDING CHILD

Simple Precautionary Measures Each year thousands of children are needlessly poisoned because adults do not take proper precautionary measures in avoiding accidental poisoning. A few simple steps can avoid a tragedy to a young child. Here are a few valuable tips on "poison proofing" your home.

● Keep handy the phone number of the poison control center nearest your home.

• Know where poison anecdotes are kept and how to properly use them.

• Keep medicines and household products out of children's sight and reach. If possible, lock them away.

• Safely discard prescription drugs no longer being taken.

• When purchasing prescription drugs always ask your pharmacist for child-proof packaging.

• When discussing drugs around children, never refer to medicines as candy or something that should be casually eaten.

• Avoid taking any medicines in the presence of children.

• It's a good idea to have syrup of ipecac in your home. This will be extremely valuable when it is necessary to induce vomiting.

Remember, always consult your doctor or poison control center before taking any action.

The Council of Family Health offers a free health aid which tells you what to do in the event of poisoning and other household emergencies.

Copies are available free by writing: Council on Family Health, 420 Lexington Avenue, New York, NY 10017.

POTATOES

When To Avoid Green potatoes contain a chemical called solanine that can cause brain and intestinal disorders, according to nutritional specialist, Carla Hughes of the University of Missouri, Columbia.

This poisonous ingredient cannot be boiled or fried away. Avoid the following:

• Potatoes that are green or bitter. Trim these affected areas away before eating.

• Avoid eating potato sprouts.

• Avoid potato stems that are green in color.

Always store potatoes in a dark place to avoid premature spoilage.

PREMENSTRUAL TENSION

Tips That May Help Premenstrual tension is the nervousness and irritability experienced by some women the week before their period. Other symptoms may include tiredness, depression, breast discomfort, temporary weight gain and bloating. Symptoms usually subside when period starts. Experts estimate about 60% of women suffer premenstraul tension.

• Reduce salt intake 2 weeks before cycle starts.
• A research study showed that simply taking 50 milligrams of vitamin B-6 daily caused an overall improvement in symptoms in 63% of the women. Foods rich in vitamin B-6 include bananas, cabbage, green leafy vegetables, whole grains and fish.

PRESCRIPTION DRUGS

Questions To Ask Your Doctor The Pharmaceutical Manufacturers Association recommends that patients ask the following questions when their doctor gives them a prescription:

• What is the medicine's name and purpose?
• What results are expected from taking it?
• How long is it necessary to wait before reporting to the doctor if there are no changes in symptoms?
• Are there any side effects?
• What side effects, if any, are supposed to be reported to the doctor? (According to a recent survey most doctors don't

143

fully explain side effects.)

- Are there any cautions to watch for while taking the medicine? Are there any foods or beverages to avoid? Other medications not to take? Any limitations on driving or other activities?
- Are there specific instructions about how and when to take the medicine?
- How long should you use the medication?
- Can the prescription be refilled? If so, are you to check with the doctor before having it refilled?

PRODUCT SAFETY

Call Toll-Free For Free Information The Consumer Product Safety Commission maintains a toll-free hotline to provide information on hazardous products. Call 1-800-638-2772 (in Maryland call 1-800-492-8104).

PROSTATE TROUBLE

Man's Most Common Affliction Prostate trouble is one of the most common afflictions of men. Medical authorities estimate that over half of the men past the age of 45 suffer some kind of prostate symptoms. At age 80 or over, as many as 95% of men suffer prostate distress. Prostate troubles can cause a variety of symtoms such as frequency of urination, getting up nights to urinate, urgency, delay in starting, abnormal retention of urine, dribbling, pain and discomfort.

Benign Prostatic Hypertrophy (BHP) This is the most common prostate problem. Simply stated, BHP is an enlargement of the prostate gland that is not cancerous. The

144

healthy prostate gland is about the size of a walnut. But enlarged, it can swell to the size of an orange. When the prostate becomes enlarged it can pinch the urethra tube causing a variety of prostate symptoms mentioned earlier.

Zinc And BPH Relief Dr. Irving Bush of Chicago's Cook County Hospital treated 19 patients who suffered from BPH. They received 34 milligrams of oral zinc a day for 2 months. After that they were placed on a long-term program of zinc dosages between 11 to 23 milligrams a day. Of the 19 patients, all reported that their painful symptoms were relieved. Five of the patients showed a decrease in prostate size. Foods rich in zinc include sea food, spinach, mushrooms, whole grains and sun flower seeds.

Complete Voiding Taking plenty of time to urinate when nature calls eased the problem of getting up nights, according to a report in the New England Journal of Medicine. Take plenty of time to void--until nothing more comes out--but don't strain. Several weeks of this training may strengthen bladder control.

Cholesterol And BPH Studies performed at Rutgers University showed a relationship between high-fat diet and BPH.

Another study reported to the American Urological Association showed there may be a connection between high cholesterol levels and prostate disease.

Another study at Metropolitan Hospital, New York, examined 100 prostates from men of all ages and found an 80% increase of cholesterol content of prostates with BPH.

See the section under heart disease for ways to reduce cholesterol levels in your body.

Prostatitis Prostatitis is an infection or inflamation of the prostate gland. Though not a serious disorder, prostatitis can be irritating and uncomfortable because it disrupts normal urination.

Zinc And Prostatitis Relief Dr. Irving Bush treated 200 patients with 11 to 34 milligrams of oral zinc per day for up to 16 weeks. Seventy percent reported a relief of symptoms. All 200 patients registered higher zinc levels. Other studies have shown that zinc has a bacteria-killing effect on the bacteria most often associated with prostate infection.

Dr. Warren Heston, PhD., Assistant Professor of Urology at the Washington University School of Medicine in St. Louis, reported that prostatic fluid of men having prostatitis had only about 1/10 the zinc of men free of this prostate trouble. Foods rich in zinc include sea food, spinach, mushrooms, whole grains and sun flower seed.

Overall Prostate Health A 10-year study covering 122,261 men aged 40 and over showed that men with a low intake of green and yellow vegetables suffered prostate cancer twice as much as those men who ate plenty of vegetables. This link between green and yellow vegetables and prostate cancer was observed in every age group, social class and region study. Scientists speculated that green and yellow vegetables are rich in vitamin A which may be responsible for the lower rate of prostate cancer.

PSORIASIS

3 Tips That May Help Psoriasis is a skin disease producing thick, red erruptions on the arms, legs or head. In severe cases it can spread throughout the entire body. Psoriasis has been evident since Biblical times. It affects between 5 to 7 percent of the population. There is no known cure for psoriasis. It also reacts erratically to treatment. One medication may help some and have no effect on others. The following measures often help:

• *Clean.* Cleaning the skin is important to prevent infection. Lotions and creams available at drug stores can

146

cleanse and reduce itching. Many of these preparations contain coal tar that helps remove scales.

● *Sun.* Many people find that regular exposure to the sun is helpful. Where sunlight is scarce a sun lamp is often used with a doctors supervision.

● *Gluten.* French researchers have found a link between psoriasis and problems in digesting gluten--a protein found in grain such as oats, barley, rye and wheat. In a preliminary study, 11 people with severe psoriasis were given a gluten-free diet. This gluten-free diet helped psorasis victims greatly.

PULSE RATE

Checking Your Pulse Rate A normal pulse rate for an adult is between 67 and 72 beats per minute when at rest. Normal pulse rate for children varies with age. The average normal pulse rate for a new born infant is about 120 beats per minute. A child's pulse rate can be anywhere from 60 to 90 beats per minute. An older child should have an average pulse rate of about 80. Normal pulse rates increase with activity, excitement and other factors.

The proper way to take a pulse rate is to place the index finger lightly on the radial artery at the wrist and count the beats for a full minute. Do not use the thumb to take the pulse rate. It may result in an inaccruate reading because the thumb has a pulse of its own.

RECTAL ITCHING

Suggestions To Relieve Itch After each bowel movement take these four steps.

1. Cleanse the rectal area with soap and warm water. Rinse

away the soap thoroughly. This procedure is much less irritating than facial tissue.

2. Sponge off the entire rectal area with rubbing alcohol. This helps kill germs and helps dry the skin.

3. Gently powder the area with talcum powder or corn starch. Powder helps the skin resist itch-producing fluids which may seep from the rectum.

4. Take a wad of cotton about half the size of a cigarette. Sprinkle it with talcum powder or corn starch. Place this cotton about ½ inch into the rectal opening--just far enough so that it will stay in place. This will soak up any seepage. If large hemorrhoids are present you may need to make the piece of cotton larger.

RELAXATION

May Increase Immunity To Disease A study performed at Ohio University showed that relaxation can cut down on stress and increase resistance to disease. Relaxation increases disease-fighting agents in the blood. These disease-fighting agents have the effects of bolstering the immune system against disease. Stress has the opposite effect on the body.

Simple Way To Relax Close your eyes and breathe in slowly. As you inhale say to yourself--I AM. Then exhale slowly saying--RELAXED. Feel your entire body loosen up and become free of tension. Repeat until you feel more relaxed.

RESISTANCE TO DISEASE

Older Persons And Zinc Supplementing the diet with zinc may help the elderly increase resistance to disease,

148

according to the results of a study by researchers at the University of California, San Diego, School of Medicine, and VA Medical Center in La Jolla, California. The study found that the equivalent of 100 milligrams of zinc a day doubled the number of antibody-producing cells in subjects whose ages ranged from 66 to 85. Antibodies are generally considered the body's first line of defense against disease.

The recommended daily requirement for zinc is 15 milligrams per day. However, the average daily zinc in the North American diet is estimated at below 15 milligrams. Foods rich in zinc include sea food, spinach, mushrooms, whole grains and sun flower seeds.

REYES SYNDROME

Preventing Problems Reyes syndrome is a rare, but often fatal disease that may follow flu or chicken pox. It occurs mostly in younger children but can also affect teenagers.

Reyes syndrome often strikes when the flu or chicken pox victim seems to be recovering. The symptoms include violent headache, persistent vomiting, lethargy and sleepiness, beligerance, disorientation and delerium.

Reyes Syndrome and Aspirin--A Possible Link The cause of Reyes Syndrome is not known but some studies suggest a possible link between the development of Reyes Syndrome and use of aspirin in flu or chicken pox.

Manufacturers of aspirin are now voluntarily putting a warning on labels which says that a physician should be consulted before aspirin is given to children, including teenagers, who have flu or chicken pox.

As a parent, if you feel you must do something while your child has the flu or chicken pox, check with your doctor to see what he recommends.

ROACHES

Killing With Boric Acid Cockroaches can contaminate your home with germs and promote disease. To kill cockroaches, sprinkle boric acid into moldings and crevices in the kitchen. This is a time-proven remedy that will kill roaches within 6 days. Roaches will not develop a resistance to boric acid as they do with commercial products. Boric acid is safer than commercial products. It is not toxic to children. It is not absorbed into the skin and not easily inhaled.

ROMANCE

2 Key Ways Women Start Romances Romance can be good for your mental health. It can reduce stress and promote relaxation. Women start almost all romances, says researcher Dr. Heather Remoff. Women use two main ways of initiating a romance.

- The woman arranges to be near a man. For example, at work a woman could arrange to be by a man during a coffee break or during lunch.
- Women also use signals to let men know they are interested in them. These signals can take the form of fluttering of the eyes and movements of the body.

SALT

Cutting Down On Your Intake Americans consume over 5.5 pounds of salt per year. Many doctors are recommending reducing salt intake as part of a program for better health.
- *Salt Shaker.* Researchers at a University studied over

2,000 diners using salt shakers with holes of various sizes. The study showed that persons using the shakers with smaller holes used less salt. The study was conducted by the University of South Wales in Sidney, Australia.

- *Lemon Juice As Salt.* A research study published in the Journal of The American Dietetic Association indicated that volunteers could not tell the difference between tomato juice seasoned with lemon juice (or citric acid) and salt.

- *Herbs As Salt.* Try replacing salt with a blend of herbs. Combine oregano, onion powder, garlic, basil, bay leaf and pepper.

- *Find Out Salt Content.* Find out the salt content of any food by calling a toll-free number established by the Sodium Information Center. Dial 1-800-622-DASH between the hours of 10:00 a.m. and 8:00 p.m., Monday through Friday, Eastern time.

SECOND OPINION (SURGERY)

Avoiding Unnecessary Surgery When you are considering surgery (that is not an emergency) you should get a second opinion, says the Federal Government's Department of Health and Human Services.

There are differences of opinion about medical problems. One doctor may recommend surgery. Another may tell you to wait. Another may recommend some other form of treatment. When you get a second opinion you get more information and increase your chances of making the right decision.

Questions You Should Ask
1. What does the doctor say is the matter with you?
2. What is the operation the doctor plans to do?
3. What are the likely benefits to you of the operation?
4. What are risks of the surgery and how likely are they to occur?

Self-diagnosis can be dangerous. If you have a serious health problem, see your doctor promptly.

5. How long would the recovery period be and what is involved?

6. What are the costs of the operation? Will your insurance cover all of those costs?

7. What will happen if you don't have the operation?

8. Are there other ways to treat your condition that could be tried first?

How To Find A Specialist To Give You A Second Opinion

1. Ask your doctor to give you the name of another doctor to see. Most doctors will encourage you to seek a second opinion. It is standard medical practice.

2. Contact your local medical society or medical schools in your area. Ask for the names of doctors specializing in problems like your's.

3. If you're under Medicare, call your local Social Security office. If you're on Medicaid call your local Welfare office for a referral.

Toll-free Hotline For Second (Or Third) Opinion Referral The Federal Government operates a free referral service that can help you locate a specialist near your home. Simply call 1-800-492-6603.

Getting Your Second Opinion Ask your doctor to send your medical records to the second doctor. By doing this you may be able to avoid the time and cost of repeating tests that have already been done.

When getting a second opinion tell the doctor:
• The name of the surgical procedure recommended.
• Any tests you know you have had.

If the second doctor agrees that surgery is the best way to treat your problem, he will refer you back to the first doctor. If he disagrees, you have to decide what to do. You could discuss the matter with the first doctor, or get a third opinion.

Medicare Pays For A Second Opinion Most state medicare programs and private insurance companies will pay for a second opinion.

SHINGLES

Speeding Up Relief Shingles is an outbreak of blisters on reddened skin. It is a highly painful condition. Shingles is caused by the same virus that causes chicken pox. It generally strikes persons over 50. About half of the U.S. population will get shingles. One shingles attack usually gives the victim immunity against another attack.

- *Vitamin E.* A study published in Archives of Dermatology showed that patients who received about 400 milligrams daily of vitamin E and who applied vitamin E to the sores directly showed an improvement.
- *Vitamin B-12 and C.* Some shingles sufferers have reported some success by taking large doses of vitamin B-12. Others report supplements of vitamin C helped overcome this condition.

SINUS CONGESTION

Suggestions For Preventing Flareups Sinus congestion is due to an inflamation of the mucus membranes that line sinus cavities. Sinus congestion can be triggered by anything that prevents mucus from draining properly. Possibilities include allergies, colds or flu, abscessed teeth, emotional stress, swimming and diving without nose plugs. Sinus congestion is often caused by a bacterial infection in the sinus cavities. Common symptoms are headache and tenderness in the forehead above and behind the eyes. Millions of Americans complain of sinus problems. Here are some rules to follow to avoid problems:

- Avoid substances you're allergic to.
- Avoid abrupt temperature changes. For example, wear a sweater in an air-conditioned room and dress warmly when you go outside on a cold day.

- Avoid household aerosol sprays. They can trigger a sinus attack. Also avoid scented hand soaps, tissue paper and perfumes.
- Smoke can trigger a sinus problem. Avoid smokey rooms. Keep your oven clean. Also keep burners clean. They can send smoke throughout the house.
- Have regular dental checkups. Tooth infections can easily spread into the sinuses causing problems.

3 Tips For Relieving Sinus Congestion
- Inhale steam from a vaporizer, especially in dry climates.
- Apply ice pack to bridge of nose and across cheek bones. This shrinks inflamed tissues, says Dr. Nicholas Murray from the University of Melbourne in Australia.
- When sinus congestion is caused by sinusitis, a bacterial infection, you should visit your doctor for treatment.

Salt Water For Sinus Congestion To relieve sinus congestion thoroughly dissolve one rounded teaspoon of table salt into one pint of warm, distilled water. (Using distilled water is important. Tap water contains chlorine and other contaminants which may be irritating to sinuses.) Cup the solution into the palm of your hand. Hold it to the nose and breathe in. Tip the head backwards so the solution can be drawn into the throat then spit out the solution.

Vitamin A An article published in Nutritional Support of Medical Practice indicates that vitamin A may actually thin mucus membranes. A lack of vitamin A may contribute to sinus congestion by hardening the membranes. Even a minor deficiency may trigger problems. Vitamin A is responsible for production of mucus-producing cells. Foods rich in vitamin A include broccoli, carrots, fish, green and yellow fruits and low-fat milk.

Heat And Water To clear sinus congestion apply hot towels to sinus area for 1 or 2 hours, 4 times a day, says Dr. Bryon Baily from Galvaston, Texas. Also, drink plenty of water to clear out congestion.

Massaging Away Sinus Headache Massaging the temple and forehead above the eyes will help relax facial nerves. This relieves tightly drawn areas of the face and brings relief to sinus and eye discomfort, according to Dr. L. L. Schneider, author of "Old Fashioned Health Remedies".

Free Sinus Information For a free pamphlet on sinus pain, write to: Sinusitis, Building #1, National Institutes of Health, 9000 Rockville Pike, Bethesda, MD 20892.

SKIN

Tips For General Care The skin is the largest body organ covering and protecting tissues, bones and organs. The skin is exposed--it's first to take abuse from the outside world. Because of this, the skin is subject to many disorders. The skin reveals the age of the body. The following recommendations will help keep skin youthful:

• Avoid harsh soaps and abrasive cleansers, advises Dr. Albert Kligman, Professor of Dermatology at the School of Medicine at the University of Pennsylvania in Philadelphia.
• Use a good moisturizer regularly.
• Avoid facial exercises, they stretch the skin. That can cause wrinkles. The less you move your face the better.
• Avoid going in the sun as much as possible. It is especially important to avoid midday sun.
• If you cannot avoid being in the sun use a sun screen. The sun can damage your skin permanently. A severe skin burn may take 15 or 20 years to show up. That's when wrinkles and sagging skin starts.
• Avoid smoking. Cigarette smoke destroys the small blood vessels in your skin which cause it to age.
• For oily skin use toners and astringents. Use during the day whenever skin gets too oily.

- Never use toners or astringents on dry skin.
- Use a hat or visor to block out the suns rays. This is especially important with sensitive skin.

Keep Skin Healthy In The Winter Winters are particularly harsh on your skin. Cold weather outside affects skin one way and heating conditions inside another. Here are some tips for winter skin care:

- Drink at least six glasses of liquid a day.
- Use a skin protector plus a moisturizer. One of the best protectors found in many skin care products is dimethicone. The best moisturizer is urea and a glyul compound. Also, use a moisturizer for your lips.
- Dampen and tone your skin twice a day.
- Properly care for hidden areas of your skin like elbows and heels. Cleanse with a gentle scrub once a week. Then apply a moisturizing cream.
- Don't forget about caring for your throat and upper chest. These areas usually get the same exposure as the face.
- Avoid extreme changes in temperature. Before coming outdoors, stop and take a minute to warm your cheeks and nose with your hands. This will help avoid risk of broken capillaries caused by abrupt temperature changes.

SLEEP

Tips For Getting A Good Nights Sleep
- Drink a glass of warm milk before going to bed.
- A warm bath or shower helps induce relaxation. Taking a warm bath or shower has the opposite effect of taking a cold shower to wake you up in the morning, says Dr. L. L. Schneider, author of "Old Fashioned Health Remedies".
- Avoid drinking coffee or any other stimulants several hours before retiring.

- Reduce salt intake. One research study showed high salt intake interfered with normal sleep.
- Avoid alcohol before bedtime. Studies show alcohol interferes with normal sleep cycles. It also depresses normal dream cycles.
- Go to bed only when tired. If you don't fall asleep in a short while, get up again until you feel tired.

Relieving Tension Before Bed Tension is a common cause of insomnia. You have a better chance of getting a good night's sleep if you can relieve tension. This simple exercise can help.

- Reach as high as possible.
- Hold this position while standing on tip-toes with fingers outreached as if reaching for the ceiling. Count to 30.
- Slowly tighten the muscles of the arms, neck, chest, abdomen, hips and legs as if holding onto an invisible object.
- Retain this position bringing yourself downward to a squatting position.
- Press on the floor with hands. Count to 30.
- Let go. Shake the arms and legs. Then retire and enjoy a good night's sleep. Repeat exercise if necessary.

Sleep And Tryptophan One of the best natural sleep aids is available at most health food stores. It's called tryptophan--an all-natural amino acid. Taking typtophan before going to bed may shorten the length of time it takes to fall asleep, says Dr. Ernest Hartmann, Professor at Tufts University School of Medicine. Subjects given one gram of tryptophan fell asleep 30-50 minutes faster than subjects who did not take tryptophan.

The amino acid tryptophan converts to serotonin in the body. Increased serotonin levels help induce sleep. Vitamins B-6 and C are necessary for the conversion of tryptophan to serotonin say researchers.

SMOKING

Greater Heart Attack Risks For Women Medical experts estimate that about 340,000 Americans die each year as a result of cigarette smoking. Smoking has been associated with heart disease, cancer, emphysema and other ailments. Despite this millions of Americans continue to smoke.

Women under 50 who smoke heavily are 7 times more likely to have a heart attack than non-smokers. When taking the birth control pill they have an even higher risk of heart attack.

Depletion Of Vitamin C Every cigarette depletes the body of about 25 milligrams of vitamin C. Some researchers say that heavy smokers need at least 140 milligrams of vitamin C a day.

What Happens When You Quit The moment you quit smoking your body starts to benefit, according to the American Cancer Society.

- Within 20 minutes your blood pressure and pulse rate drop to normal, and oxygen level of blood increases to normal.
- After 24 hours your chance of heart attack decreases.
- After 48 hours your ability to smell and taste improves.
- After 72 hours bronchial tubes relax making breathing easier. Lung capacity also increases.
- After 2 weeks to 3 months your circulation improves and lung function increases up to 30 percent.
- From 1 to 9 months after quitting coughing, sinus congestion, fatigue and shortness of breath decrease. Your overall body energy level increases.
- After 5 years lung cancer death rate decreases. (Tobacco contains 30 cancer causing agents.)
- After 10 years lung cancer death rate drops to 12 deaths per 100,000--almost the same rate of non-smokers. Pre-cancerous cells are replaced. The risk of other cancers such as

158

mouth, larynx, esophagus, bladder, kidney and pancreas also decrease.

15 Suggestions For Cutting Down On Cigarette Smoking The National Cancer Insitute recommends the following:

- Smoke only half of each cigarette.
- Each day, postpone lighting your first cigarette one hour.
- Decide you will smoke only during odd or even hours of the day.
- Decide beforehand how many cigarettes you'll smoke during the day. For each additional smoke, give a dollar to your favorite charity.
- Don't smoke when you first experience a craving. Wait several minutes; and during this time, change your activity or talk to someone.
- Stop buying cigarettes by the carton. Wait until one pack is empty before buying another.
- Stop carrying cigarettes with you at home and at work. Make them difficult to get to.
- Smoke only under circumstances which are not especially pleasurable for you. If you like to smoke with others, smoke alone.
- Make yourself aware of each cigarette by using the opposite hand, or putting cigarettes in an unfamiliar location or different pocket to break the automatic reach.
- If you light up many times during the day without even thinking about it, try to look in a mirror each time you put a match to your cigarette--you may decide you don't need it.
- Don't smoke "automatically." Smoke only those you really want.
- Reward yourself in some way other than smoking.
- Reach for a glass of juice instead of a cigarette for a "pick-me-up."
- Change your eating habits to aid in cutting down. For example, drink milk, which is frequently considered incompatible with smoking. End meals or snacks with

something which won't lead to a cigarette.

- Don't empty your ashtrays. This will not only remind you of how many cigarettes you have smoked each day, the sight and smell of stale butts will be very unpleasant.

Quitting Smoking--The First Day On the day you decide to quit smoking do the following, says the National Cancer Institute:

- Throw away all cigarettes and matches. Hide lighters and ashtrays.
- Visit the dentist and have your teeth cleaned to get rid of tobacco stains. Notice how nice they look, and resolve to keep them that way.
- Make a list of things you'd like to buy yourself or someone else. Estimate the cost in terms of packs of cigarettes, and put the money aside to buy these presents.
- Keep very busy on the big day. Go to the movies, exercise, take long walks, go bike riding.
- Buy yourself a treat or do something special to celebrate.

Immediately After Quitting

- The first few days after you quit, spend as much free time as possible in places where smoking is prohibited, e.g., libraries, museums, theaters, department stores, churches, etc.
- Drink large quantities of water and fruit juice.
- Try to avoid alcohol, coffee and other beverages with which you associate cigarette smoking.
- Strike up a conversation with someone instead of a match for a cigarette.
- If you miss the sensation of having a cigarette in your hand, play with something else--a pencil, a paper clip, a marble.
- If you miss having something in your mouth, try toothpicks or a fake cigarette.

Avoid Temptation

- Instead of smoking after meals, get up from the table and

160

brush your teeth or go for a walk.

• If you always smoke while driving, take public transportation for a while.

• Temporarily avoid situations you strongly associate with the pleasurable aspects of smoking, e.g., watching your favorite TV program, sitting in your favorite chair, having a cocktail before dinner, etc.

• Develop a clean, fresh non-smoking environment around yourself--at work and at home.

• Until you are confident of your ability to stay off cigarettes, limit your socializing to healthful, outdoor activities or situations where smoking is prohibited.

• If you must be in a situation where you'll be tempted to smoke (such as a cocktail or dinner party), try to associate with the non-smokers there.

• Look at cigarette ads more critically to better understand the attempt to make individual brands appealing.

When You Have The Urge

• Keep oral substitutes handy--things like carrots, pickles, sun-flower seeds, apples, celery, raisins, sugarless gum and so on.

• Take 10 deep breaths and hold the last one while lighting a match. Exhale slowly and blow out the match. Pretend it is a cigarette and crush it out in an ashtray.

• Take a shower or bath if possible.

• Learn to relax quickly and deeply. Make yourself limp, visualizing a soothing, pleasing situation and get away from it all for a moment. Concentrate on that peaceful image and nothing else.

• Light incense or a candle instead of a cigarette.

SNEEZING

Don't Hold A Sneeze Back Sneezing releases bacteria and viruses that can prolong your illness. Holding back a

161

sneeze may infect your sinuses and even cause ear infection, says Dr. Chole, Professor at the University of California. When you do sneeze you should sneeze with your mouth open but covered with your hand.

SNORING

4 Suggestions For Snorers
• Sleep sideways rather than on your back. Prop pillows on either side of your body to prevent rolling over on your back.
• Avoid tranquilizers or sleeping pills before bedtime.
• Tilt the bed with the head upwards. The best way is to put 6 to 8 inch wooden blocks under the front legs of the bed.
• Avoid alcoholic beverages within 2 hours of going to bed.

STIFF NECK

Relieving Discomfort Stiff necks are most often caused by a muscle cramp brought about by a chill, sleeping in a cramped position or sudden twisting movement when backing up a car. Try these suggestions for fast relief:

• Apply hot packs, or take a hot shower concentrating on sore neck area.
• Gently massage neck. A vibrator is often helpful.
• Take aspirin to relieve pain if needed.

Stiff Neck Exercise
1. While standing, let the head move slowly forward and downward without forcing it.
2. Firmly interlace the fingers behind the neck.
3. Slowly bring the head upwards as if to look at the ceiling directly above. Hold the head in this position for approximately 30 seconds.

Self-diagnosis can be dangerous. If you have a serious health problem, see your doctor promptly.

4. Relax to normal position resting 2 or 3 minutes.

5. Repeat the same procedure 6 times starting with step 1 and resting after each stretching.

Stiff Neck Rub Have your druggist mix a solution of 15% oil of Wintergreen and 85% rubbing alcohol. Apply this solution to the stiff muscles of your neck. Rub very lightly. After the area is well-coated cover it with a hot damp cloth, recommends Dr. L. L. Schneider, author of "Old Fashioned Health Remedies".

STRESS

How To Deal With Stress Stress is with us all the time. It is an unavoidable part of our lives. Stress is unique and personal to each of us. What may be stressful to one person may actually be relaxing to another. Stress can be defined as too much of the wrong sort of pressure. Too much emotional stress can cause physical illness such as high blood pressure, ulcers or even heart disease. Recognizing early signs of stress and then doing something about it can make an important difference in the quality of your life. It may actually influence your survival.

How The Body Reacts To Stress To use stress in a positive way and prevent it from becoming distress, you should become aware of your own reactions to stressful events. The body responds to stress by going through three stages: (1) alarm, (2) recovery, and (3) exhaustion.

Let's take the example of a typical commuter in rush-hour traffic. If a car suddenly pulls out in front of him, his initial alarm reaction may include fear of an accident, anger at the driver who committed the action, and general frustration. His body may respond in the alarm stage by releasing hormones into the bloodstream which cause his face to flush, perspiration to form, his stomach to have a sinking feeling,

163

and his arms and legs to tighten. The next stage is recovery, in which the body repairs damage caused by the stress. If the stress of driving continues with repeated close calls or traffic jams, however, his body will not have time to make repairs. He may become so conditioned to expect potential problems when he drives that he tightens up at the beginning of ech commuting day. Eventually, he may even develop one of the diseases of stress, such as migraine headaches, high blood pressure, backaches or insomnia. While it is impossible to live completely free of stress and distress, it is possible to prevent some distress as well as to minimize its impact when it can't be avoided.

Helping Yourself When stress does occur, it is important to recognize and deal with it. Here are some suggestions for ways to handle stress. As you begin to understand more about how stress affects you as an individual, you will come up with your own ideas of helping to ease the tensions.

● *Try Physical Activity.* When you are nervous, angry or upset, release the pressures through exercise or physical activity. Running, walking, playing tennis or working in your garden are just some of the activities you might try. Physical exercise will relieve that "up tight" feeling, relax you and turn the frowns into smiles. Remember, your body and your mind work together.

● *Share Your Stress.* It helsp to talk to someone about your concerns and worries. Perhaps a friend, family member, teacher or counselor can help you see your problem in a different light. If you feel your problem is serious, you might seek professional help from a psychologist, psychiatrist or social worker. Knowing when to ask for help may avoid more serious problems later.

● *Know Your Limits.* If a problem is beyond your control and cannot be changed at the moment, don't fight the situation. Learn to accept what is--for now--until such time when you can change it. Learn how to say no to demands that overburden you.

• **Take Care Of Yourself.** You are special. Get enough rest and eat well. If you are irritable and tense from lack of sleep or if you are not eating correctly, you will have less ability to deal with stressful situations. If stress repeatedly keeps you from sleeping, you should ask your doctor for help.

• **Make Time For Fun.** Schedule time for both work and recreation. Play can be just as important to your well-being as work; you need a break from your daily routine to just relax and have fun.

• **Be a participant.** One way to keep from getting bored, sad and lonely is to go where it's all happening. Sitting alone can make you feel frustrated. Instead of feeling sorry for yourself, get involved and become a participant. Offer your services in neighborhood volunteer organizations. Help yourself by helping other people. Get involved in the world and the people around you, and you'll find they will be attracted to you. You're on your way to making new friends and enjoying new activities.

• **Check Off Your Tasks.** Trying to take care of everything at once can seem overwhelming, and, as a result, you may not accomplish anything. Instead, make a list of what tasks you have to do, then do one at a time, checking them off as they're completed. Give priority to the most important ones and do those first.

• **Must You Always Be Right?** Do other people upset you-- particularly when they don't do things your way? Try cooperation instead of confrontation; it's better than fighting and always being "right." A little give and take on both sides will reduce the strain and make you both feel more comfortable.

• **It's O.K. To Cry.** A good cry can be a healthy way to bring relief to your anxiety, and it might even prevent a headache or other physical consequence. Take some deep breaths; they also release tension.

• **Create A Quiet Scene.** You can't always run away, but you can "dream the impossible dream." A quiet country scene painted mentally, or on canvas, can take you out of the turmoil of a stressful situation. Change the scene by reading a good book or playing beautiful music to create a sense of peace and tranquility.

• *Avoid Self-Medication.* Although you can use drugs to relieve stress temporarily, drugs do not remove the conditions that caused the stress in the first place. Drugs, in fact, may be habit-forming and create more stress than they take away. They should be taken only on the advice of your doctor.

The Art Of Relaxation The best strategy for avoiding stress is to learn how to relax. Unfortunately, many people try to relax at the same pace that they lead the rest of their lives. For a while, tune out your worries about time, productivity, and "doing right." You will find satisfaction in just *being*, without striving. Find activities that give you pleasure and that are good for your mental and physical well-being. Forget about always winning. Focus on relaxation, enjoyment and health. *Be good to yourself.*

Nutritional Considerations Excessive amounts of stress can deplete your body of essential nutrients, thereby weakening your coping abilities.

B-complex Vitamins. B-complex vitamins help maintain the health of your nervous system. Even a slight vitamin B deficiency can cause irritability and depression.

Vitamin B-1 (Thiamin). Several dietary factors interfere with the ability of your body to utilize thiamin. Consuming sugar raises thiamin requirements. Thiamin is affected by tannic acid, so the consumption of 4 to 6 cups of tea per day can produce symptomatic thiamin deficiency. Also, heavy alcohol consumption is known for its ability to cause a thiamin deficiency, according to a study in Nutritional Abborations and Clinical Pharmacy and Therapeutics.

Pantothenic Acid. Pantothenic acid is another B-vitamin that can improve the ability of even well-nourished people to withstand stress.

Vitamin C. During times of physical stress vitamin C needs

166

rise higher than the recommended dietary allowance. Also, infections, burns and cigarette smoking drain the tissues of vitamin C.

Magnesium. Magnesium is another nutrient drained from the body by stress. Studies indicate that a magnesium deficiency weakens the body's ability to cope with stress.

When the body is not adequately provided with complete nutrition it is more difficult for the body to recover from the physical effects of stress.

STRETCH MARKS

Try Vitamin E Many people have reported that vitamin E cream helps soften and relieve stretch marks. Also, supplementing the diet with about 400 I.U.'s of vitamin E daily helps stretch marks. Foods rich in vitamin E include dark green vegetables, fruits and rice.

STUTTERING

Help Is Available Many famous people throughout history have stuttered. They include Moses, Winston Churchill, King George VI, Charles Darwin, Thomas Jefferson, Mel Tillis and Jimmy Stewart. Experts say that stutterers are smarter than the average person, having an I.Q. about 14 points higher. Stutterers can be cured or helped considerably to control their problem. Most of the therapies involve concentration upon air flow through the vocal cords and relaxing. By doing this, stutterers are less likely to trigger muscular spasms often responsible for stuttering. Hypnosis has also shown to be a highly effective therapy for stuttering.

Stuttering Hotline To get help or information on stuttering write: National Center For Stuttering, 200 East 33rd Street, New York, NY 10016. You can also call toll-free. The number is 1-800-221-2483. The Center can give you a recommendation for professional treatment in your area.

SUGAR

4 Reasons To Cut Sugar Intake Many medical experts are recommending reduced intake of refined sugar. Here are some reasons why.

- High intake of sugar can deplete the body's supply of B vitamins, particularly vitamin B-1. This can result in poor concentration, memory problems, irritability and depression.
- Sugar produces a short-term energy boost lasting about an hour. After that your energy level plummets.
- Sugar may be habit forming. Sugar increases the production of insulin resulting in lower blood sugar levels. This can lead to a strong craving for sugar on a continual basis.
- Sugar also promotes tooth decay. The more sugar you consume, the higher your chances of getting cavities.

Sugar Substitutes Instead of sprinkling sugar over cereal or fruit, try a blend of sweet spices, such as cinnamon, nutmeg, cloves, allspice and anise.

SUNTAN

Suggestions For Preventing Skin Damage A suntan makes you look great, but beware of the longer-term effects. Over time the sun's rays will leave your skin tough, leathery and dry, say skin experts. Crows feet around the eyes are often caused by squinting under bright sunlight. Prevent damage to your skin by following some simple rules:

• Avoid peak hours of sunshine between 10 a.m. and 2 p.m This is when ultraviolet rays are the strongest.

• Limit your exposure to the sun. Depending on your type of skin, you should begin with only 15 minutes in the sun. Use sun tan lotions that contain sun screen. Sun screens range from a strength of 2 to 15. These sun protection factors (SPF) give you an idea how long you can stay in the sun without burning. For example, if you could normally stay in the sun 15 minutes without burning a lotion with a SPF of 2 would allow you to stay in the sun 30 minutes. Here is the meaning of the various sun protection factors.

1. SPF 2 to 4: Minimal protection from sun burning. Permits suntanning. Recommended for people who rarely burn and tan easily.

2. SPF 4 to 6: Moderate protection from sunburning. Permits some suntanning. Recommended for people who tan with minimal burning.

3. SPF 6 to 8: Extra protection from sunburning. Permits limited suntanning. Recommended for people who burn moderately and tan gradually.

4. SPF 8 to under 15: Maximal protection from sunburning. Permits little or no suntanning. Recommended for people who always burn easily and tan minimally.

5. SPF 15 or greater: Ultra protection from sunburn. Offers the most protection. Permits no suntanning. Recommended for people who burn easily and never tan.

• Apply lotion all over your body. Make sure you have enough lotion on sensitive areas such as the nose, lips and shoulders.

• Try to avoid squinting your eyes while in the sun. The tiny lines around your eyes commonly called "crows feet" can be caused by squinting.

• Remember that the sun's rays penetrate water about 3

feet below the surface. So don't think you are not being exposed to the sun because you're under water.

- In high altitudes air is less dense and burning rays are more intense. This means you are more likely to burn.

- When you've had enough sun but are not ready to leave, cover up with clothing. That will block out the sun's rays.

- After exposure to the sun take a warm shower, then smooth on a moisturizing cream or lotion.

SUPPORT (Self Help) GROUPS

Where To Find Help There are support groups to help you or your family cope with any type of medical, health or psychological problem. Throughout the United States there are an estimated 500,000 support groups serving about 15 million people. Some are highly structured like Alcoholics Anonymous. Others are informal. Meetings are held in the homes of members. Some groups work closely with health professionals. Others go it alone. All self help groups share a common goal: the bringing together of those having similar problems and, through sharing, gain strength and support from each other. Many groups keep current on the latest medical research. They find out about treatment breakthroughs before many medical doctors.

There are two National Clearinghouse Organizations which provide information about local support groups in your area. Their addresses are:

SELF-HELP CENTER
1600 Dodge Avenue
Evanston, IL 60201

THE NATIONAL SELF-HELP CLEARING HOUSE
Dept. N85
Cuny Graduate Center
33 W. 42nd St., Room 1227
New York, NY 10036

SWALLOWING PILLS AND CAPSULES

The Best Way To Swallow

• *Tablets.* A tablet should be placed in the mouth with a small amount of water. The head should be tilted backward and the tablet or pill swallowed, says Dr. Ace Brown of Doctors Hospital in Augusta, Georgia.

• *Capsules.* A capsule should be placed in your mouth with a small sip of water. Then tip your head or upper part of your body forward. This will cause the capsule to float toward the back of the mouth where it can be swallowed easily.

TEETH, SENSITIVE

The Cause About 1 in every 4 adults experience painful discomfort of sensitive teeth. This can occur when the natural, protective tooth covering wears away or when the gums surrounding the root of the tooth recede. As a result, the root surface becomes exposed making it extra sensitive to heat and cold, causing discomfort and pain.

New Tooth Paste For Sensitive Teeth In controlled clinical studies, many people using a tooth paste called Denquel reported significant relief after two weeks of regular use. After four weeks, 90 percent reported relief of sensitivity. To obtain maximum relief it is important to brush at least two times a day or as your dentist directs. If you brush infrequently or stop brushing once the pain is reduced, sensitivity could return. Denquel is pleasent-tasting and is available at most drug stores.

TEETH AND GUMS

3 Tips To Keep Them Healthy
• Use a floride toothpaste.
• Use unwaxed dental floss between teeth and below gum line.
• Use a water irrigating device to stimulate and thoroughly clean your gums, according to the American Dental Association.

TEMPERATURE

Finding Your Normal Temperature The body temperature for a normal adult is 98.6 when the thermometer is placed under the tongue. When the temperature is taken through the rectum, the temperature is about 1 degree higher.

Temperatures can vary from 98.6 and still be normal. To find out your normal temperature, take it when you are feeling well. Then the next time you are sick you can measure the variation from normal.

Oral Temperature Oral temperature should not be taken after you have had a cold drink or brushed your teeth. Wait fifteen to thirty minutes. Then follow these basic steps.

1. Wash your hands and rinse the thermometer in cool water.
2. Holding the thermometer by the top (not the bulb end) shake it with a quick snap of the wrist until the mercury goes down to 96 degrees fahrenheit or lower.
3. Place the bulb end of the thermometer well under the tongue and keep the mouth closed (without biting) for at least 3 minutes. Young children and elderly patients should not be left alone with a fever thermometer in place.
4. Remove the thermometer and rotate it until the mercury level can be seen. A good light helps but don't hold the

thermometer close to a lamp. The heat could affect the reading.

Rectal Temperature Follow these basic steps:

1. Wash your hands and rinse the thermometer in cool water.

2. Holding the thermometer by the top, shake it with a quick snap of the wrist until the mercury goes to 96 degrees fahrenheit or lower.

3. Lubricate the thermometer with a lubricant such as vaseline.

4. Have the patient lie on one side and breathe through the mouth. Infants and small children may be on their sides, backs or tummies. Separate the buttocks with your free hand and gently insert the thermometer almost half an inch into the rectum. Leave it, or hold it in place, especially in infants and toddlers, for about 4 minutes.

5. Remove, wipe off the lubricant and read it like an oral thermometer. Rectal temperatures are about 1 degree higher than oral readings.

6. After use, wash the thermometer in cool, soapy water. Never wash in warm or hot water and do not store near heat.

TENDONITIS

Suggestions For Tendonitis Discomfort Tendonitis is an inflammation of the tissues that connect muscles to the bone. It is common in people over 30. Tendonitis can be caused by sudden stress or prolonged activity. It most often affects the hand, shoulder, ankle, knee or hip.

• Give the affected area a period of rest until pain subsides.

• Apply ice to the affected area three or four times a day for periods of up to 20 minutes.

• After about two days replace the ice treatments with heat

treatments. The heat treatments can be hot packs, heating pads or hot showers.

Preventing Tendonitis Taking time to warm up before physical activity is a simple way to prevent tendonitis. For example, calf and leg muscle stretching before jogging may help prevent tendonitis in the Achilles tendon.

TENSION

Suggestions To Help You Relax
- Sit quietly in a comfortable position.
- Close your eyes.
- Relax all your muscles beginning at your feet and progressing up to your face.
- Do this twice daily.

Quick Tension-Relief Method Your eyes use ¼ of the nervous energy consumed by the body, says Dr. Edmund Jacobson of the University of Chicago. Relaxing the eyes can help relax the entire body.

Try this simple, quick method. Lean back and close your eyes. Then silently say to your eyes let go. Stop frowning. Stop straining. Let go. Let go. Repeat for at least one minute.

TERMITES

Store Wood Away From Home Do not store firewood within 30 feet of your home. Firewood can be a prime source of termites which can infest your home and weaken the foundation. This is also true with storing other wood products near your home.

Self-diagnosis can be dangerous. If you have a serious health problem, see your doctor promptly.

THROAT, SORE

5 Tips To Reduce Discomfort
• Gargle with warm salt water every 2 hours for about 5 minutes (1 teaspoon salt per 8 ounce glass of warm water).
• Drink plenty of water or juices (about 8 ounces per hour).
• Take aspirin for mild fever and discomfort.
• Suck lozenges to help relieve pain.
• Don't smoke or be in a smoky room.

When To Call The Doctor
• Sore throat continues for 5 days.
• Fever over 101.
• Rash develops.
• You have history of rheumatic fever or kidney disease.

Your Toothbrush A study in Medical World News reported that bacteria living on your toothbrush can cause lingering throat infections. It takes only 17 to 35 days for a toothbrush to become heavily infected. If you have recurring, minor sore throats try changing your toothbrush about every 2 weeks.

THUNDER STORMS

Preventing Being Struck By Lightning When a thunder storm threatens, here are some tips to avoid being struck by lightning.

• Get inside a house, building, or metal vehicle that is not a convertible.
• If you cannot reach a building or car do not stand under a tall, isolated tree.
• Do not stand above the surrounding landscape like a hill top. Avoid open fields or the beach. Avoid open water if in a small boat.

• Stay away from metal equipment, wire fences, clothes lines, metal pipes and other metal objects that would attract lightning to you.

• If in a forest go to a low area under a thick growth of small trees.

TICS

Ridding Your Pet Of Tics
• Using a cotton swab dab alcohol on the tic. As the tic reacts by releasing itself from your pet's skin grasp the tic with your thumb and forefinger, twist and yank out.

• If long hair prevents getting at the tic apply margarine or vegetable shortening to the tic, then follow the directions above.

TOOTHACHE

What To Do When You Can't Call Your Dentist
• First, try flossing between teeth in the area of pain. Sometimes food particles lodged between teeth can cause discomfort.

• Try cleansing the cavity to remove food debris.

• Apply warm oil of cloves, available at a health food store or pharmacy. Pour a little in a teaspoon and heat with a match. Dab into the cavity with a toothpick or wooden match.

• For larger cavities mix the oil of cloves with zinc oxide powder to make a thick paste. Press a glob of this mixture into the cavity area with fingertips. Clean off excess with a tooth pick.

• Place a well-padded ice bag on the area of pain. Take

aspirin. (Never place aspirin in a cavity. It can cause tooth and tissue damage.)

What To Do If Crown Comes Off When a crown comes off and you are unable to get to a dentist, here's what to do. Wash the crown, dry it and put petroleum jelly into it. Then carefully reposition it over your tooth. If you do not do this and the crown is left off for a period of time, it may not be possible for your dentist to recement it because the adjacent teeth may have shifted.

Massaging Jaw Muscles Sometimes a toothache may be caused by tense, sore muscles in your jaw. The pain felt in the mouth mimics a toothache but tense jaw muscles are the real culprit. If this is the cause of your mouth pain, take the index fingers of both hands and gently massage (in a circular motion) the jaw muscles where the jaw connects. Continue this until the pain subsides. If the pain does not subside, consult your dentist if needed.

TOOTH DECAY

Cheese To Prevent Tooth Decay Certain kinds of cheese may help prevent tooth decay, says Dr. Charles Schachtele, Professor of Dentistry at the University of Minnesota. Cheeses that work best are Swiss, cheddar and monterrey jack. These cheeses prevent acid from forming on teeth and promoting decay.

Avoid Raisins A study published in the Journal of the American Dental Association says raisins are more harmful to the teeth than any other common snack, including chocolate, cookies, caramel and fudge. The report says raisins cause more cavities because they stick to your teeth.

Toothbrushes And Cavities It is a good idea to dispose of a toothbrush after about one month. After then bristles become worn and the toothbrush loses its effectiveness and may become contaminated with bacteria. A study in Medical World News reported it takes only 17 to 35 days for a toothbrush to become heavily infected. This is not surprising since a toothbrush provides a warm, moist environment for fast bacterial growth.

Citrus Fruits Citrus fruits such as lemons, oranges, grapefruit and tangerines contain citric acid which can cause damage to the enamel of your teeth. To avoid damage, rinse your mouth after eating or drinking any citrus fruit. Also avoid the habit of sucking on oranges, grapefruit or lemons.

URINARY TRACT INFECTIONS (BLADDER INFECTION)

How To Avoid About one-third of all women age 20 to 40 are likely to suffer from recurring urinary tract infections, says Dr. Rosemary Lindan of Western Reserve University. Women get urinary tract infections 10 times as often as men. Here are some tips to avoid urinary tract infections.

• Drink plenty of water--from 6 to 12 glasses a day. This will encourage frequent urination which empties the bladder and flushes out bacteria. Diluting the urine also eases urinary symptoms.

• Wipe from front to back after urinating. This will prevent moving fecal bacteria closer to the opening of the bladder. When possible clean the anal and vaginal areas with a stream of water after going to the bathroom.

• Be sure the genital area is clean before sex. Use a spermicidal germicidal lubricant during sex.

• Urinate as soon as possible after sexual intercourse to flush out bacteria. It may be necessary to drink a glass of water before sex so it's possible to urinate afterwards. This will flush out any bacteria that may have entered the bladder during sex.

• Use a water-soluable lubricant, such as vaseline if the vagina is dry. If delicate tissues are bruised they may become infected.

• Check with a gynecologist if a diaphragm may be contributing to your urinary tract infections. If so, another type of contraceptive should be used. A study in the New England Journal of Medicine showed that women who use a diaphragm have twice as many urinary tract infections as other women.

• Use tampons instead of sanitary napkins. Bacteria can more easily build up on napkins.

• Take showers instead of baths. Bacteria can easily travel up the urinary tract while you are sitting in the bathtub.

• Never use bubblebath. It's irritating and can make you more prone to an infection.

• Avoid wearing tight slacks or jeans. Tight clothing contributes to urinary tract bacteria growth.

• Wear cotton panties. They are more absorbent than nylon or synthetic underwear.

• Consider whether syptoms occur after use of spermicidal creams, swimming in a chlorinated pool or bike riding.

Cranberry Juice Kills Bacteria Some doctors prescribe cranberry juice for bladder infections. Cranberry juice has a high concentration of vitamin C. Just one cup has over 100 milligrams of vitamin C. When vitamin C is in the urine it promotes health of the bladder, says Dr. Alan Gaby of Baltimore, Maryland. Vitamin C can help kill the E. coli bacteria--the most common cause of urinary tract infections.

Cranberry juice also contains hippuric acid which tends to inhibit the growth of bacteria. Another doctor recommends a

6 ounce glass of cranberry juice twice a day for urinary tract infections.

VACATIONS

What Health Care Products To Take Along
- If you wear glasses carry an extra pair with you. Also carry a copy of your prescription. This is also true if you wear contact lenses.
- Take prescriptions for all medicines that you use. For medicines you take with you be sure labels clearly indicate what the medicines are.
- Take along a nasal decongestant if you are flying in an airplane.
- Take aspirin or acetaminophen (tylenol or similar products). This is the best medication for headache or other pain.
- For diarrhea effective medications are Lomotil and Imodium.
- For constipation take along Milk of Magnesia tablets or Ex-Lax. Don't let more than 2 days go by without a bowel movement.
- For infection the best thing to use is Tetracycline. It is especially effective for throat infections. Tetracycline is available only through a doctor's prescription.
- For an acid stomach take along Gelusel, Maalox or Tums.
- For motion sickness take dramamine. Another natural preparation for motion sickness is ginger root. Ginger root is available at most health food stores. Ginger root is sometimes better than dramamine because it does not cause drowsiness.
- For trouble sleeping you should carry sleeping pills or tranquilizers. These are best obtained from your doctor. Tryptophan tablets available at a health food store are a good natural sleep aid.
- For sitting out in the sun be sure to take a sun screen.

VENEREAL DISEASE

Call Toll-Free For Free Information This is a little-known service provided by the Federal government. You can get free, confidential and anonymous information on all aspects of sexually-transmitted diseases. You can get free consultation and referral information. Call 1-800-982-5883 (in Pennsylvania call 1-800-462-4966).

VITAMIN OVERDOSE

More Is Not Always Better In fact, taking too much of some vitamins can cause health problems over time. This is because some vitamins (fat-soluable) accumulate in your body and are not eliminated. Over time this accumulation in the body can cause you problems.

Vitamin A Vitamin A can produce toxic symptoms when 5 to 8 times the Recommended Daily Allowance (RDA) is consumed over a long period of time. The RDA for vitamin A is 5,000 I.U.'s. These toxic symptoms may include headache, blurred vision, impaired eyesight and flaking of the skin. It's a good idea to get vitamin A from beta-carotene supplements. With beta-carotene the body absorbs only the vitamin A that is needed.

Vitamin D Taking too much vitamin D over time can cause weakness, loss of appetite, nausea, body aches and stiffness. Overdose of vitamin D increases absorption of calcium. This excess calcium may be deposited in the heart, lungs, kidneys and even the brain. These calcium deposits can cause organ damage.

Vitamin B-6 Taking daily supplements of vitamin B-6 of 200 mgs. for over a month can cause convulsions.

Vitamin B-1 Megadoses of vitamin B-1 can cause bad breath.

WARTS

Safe Wart Remover According to a panel of medical experts working for the U.S. Food and Drug Administration (FDA), only one over-the-counter ingredient is both safe and effective in removing warts. That ingredient is salicylic acid, available in many drug store preparations. Salicylic acid gets rid of the wart by destroying the outer surface so it can be peeled away. FDA officials warn not to use salicylic acid in the following cases:

- If you are a diabetic or have poor circulation.
- Don't use on warts that have hair growing out of them, genital warts or warts on the face or mucus membranes. Don't use on moles or birthmarks.
- Discontinue use if excessive irritation occurs.
- Don't use near the eyes.

Vitamin E For Warts Many persons report that applying 28,000 I.U.'s of vitamin E to a wart, one or two times daily helps them go away. Also take 400 I.U.'s of vitamin E daily.

WATERBEDS

Possible Danger For Babies Waterbeds are great for adults, but might spell trouble for a baby. A baby may not be able to turn over on the water bed and as a result could suffocate. Don't let a baby lie face down on a water bed. It's a good idea to always supervise a baby on a water bed.

WINE

May Help You Relax A glass of wine before or after dinner can often help you relax, say medical experts.

Inexpensive wines can be just as good as expensive wines. For example, in a test of 160 wines and champaigns judges found that inexpensive wines were hard to tell from expensive wines. Experts say an $8.00 bottle of Paul Masson from California was judged better than a French rose' costing $30.00. A $5.00 Spanish wine was judged as good as a French wine costing $60.00.

WORKING WOMEN

Have Unhappier Marriages Wives who work are much less satisfied with their marriages than housewives, says Dr. Harold Voth, Professor at the University of Kansas. Working wives have more complaints about their mates and tend to respect them less. Working wives often resent their paychecks going for household necessities. They would rather spend their earnings on something else.

WORLD-WIDE HEALTH FORECAST

Finding Out About Health Risks If you plan a trip anyplace in the world it is a good idea to call ahead to find out if there are any health problems present in the country you plan to visit. Many health problems can crop up quickly causing the traveler undue exposure to potentially hazardous diseases.

Toll-Free Hotline Before going on a trip call the World Wide Health Forecast. The number is 1-800-368-3531. This hotline will give you the latest news on medical conditions in countries around the world.

SECTION II

OTHER
IMPORTANT
HEALTH INFORMATION

Who's Who in Health Care

General Care

Doctors of medicine (M.D.) use all accepted methods of medical care. They treat diseases and injuries, provide preventive care, do routine checkups, prescribe drugs, and do some surgery. M.D.'s complete medical school plus 3 to 7 years of graduate medical education. They must be licensed by the state in which they practice.

Doctors of osteopathic medicine (D.O.) also provide general health care to individuals and families. The training they receive is similar to that of an M.D. In addition to drugs, surgery, and other treatments, a D.O. may manipulate muscles and bones to treat specific problems.

Internists (M.D.) are M.D.'s or D.O.'s who specialize in the diagnosis and medical treatment of diseases in adults. Internists do not perform surgery or deliver babies.

Family practitioners (M.D.) are M.D.'s or D.O.'s who specialize in providing comprehensive health care for all members of a family, on a continuing basis, regardless of age or sex.

The above doctors might refer patients to a number of medical specialists including:

- Cardiologist--a heart specialist.
- Dermatologist--a skin specialist.
- Endocrinologist--a specialist in disorders of the glands of internal secretion, such as diabetes.
- Gastroenterologist--a specialist in diseases of the digestive tract.
- Gynecologist--a specialist in the female reproductive system.
- Neurologist--a specialist in disorders of the nervous system.

- Oncologist--a specialist in tumors and cancer.
- Ophthalmologist--an eye specialist.
- Rheumatologist--a specialist in arthritis and rheumatism.
- Urologist--a specialist in the urinary system, including the bladder and kidneys in both sexes and the male reproductive system.

Most of the services of M.D.'s, D.O.'s or specialists who have M.D. or D.O. degrees normally are covered by Medicare.

Physician assistants (P.A.) most often work in doctors' offices or hospitals doing some of the tasks traditionally performed by doctors. They do physical examinations, take medical histories, carry out diagnostic tests and develop treatment plans for patients. Their education includes 2 to 4 years of college followed by a 2-year period of specialized training. P.A.'s must always work under the supervision of a doctor but, depending on state laws, the supervision can be by telephone rather than in person. In some states P.A.'s can prescribe certain drugs. Medicare will only pay for the services provided by a P.A. if they are performed in a hospital or doctor's office under the supervision of a doctor.

Nurse practitioners (R.N., N.P.) are registered nurses with training beyond basic nursing education. Nurse practitioners perform physical examinations and diagnostic tests, counsel patients and develop treatment programs. Regulations regarding their duties vary from state to state. Nurse practitioners may work independently, such as in rural clinics or may be staff members at hospitals and other health facilities. Medicare will help pay for services performed under the supervision of a doctor.

Registered nurses (R.N.) may have 2, 3 or 4 years of education in a nursing school. In addition to performing bedside nursing duties, such as giving medicine, administering treatments and educating patients, R.N.'s often hold supervisory and teaching positions in hospitals, long-term care facilities and colleges. R.N.'s also work in doctors' offices, clinics and community health agencies. Medicare does not cover private duty nursing. It helps pay for general nursing services by reimbursing hospitals, skilled nursing facilities and home health agencies for part of the nurses' salaries.

Registered dietitians (R.D.) provide nutritional care and dietary counseling. Most of them work in hospitals or doctors' offices but some have private practices. R.D.'s complete a bachelor's degree and an internship (or an approved coordinated undergraduate program) and, in addition, pass an examination. Medicare generally will not pay for a dietitian's services. However, it does reimburse hospitals and skilled nursing facilities for a portion of dietitians' salaries.

Physical therapists (P.T.) help people whose strength, ability to move, sensation or range of motion is impaired. They may use exercise, heat, cold or water therapy; or other treatments to control pain, strengthen muscles and improve coordination. All P.T.'s complete a program leading to a bachelor's degree, and some of them receive further postgraduate training. Patients are usually referred by a doctor, and Medicare pays some of the costs of outpatient treatments. Physical therapy performed in a hospital or skilled nursing facility is covered by Medicare.

Occupational therapists (O.T.) assist patients with handicaps to function more independently. They may provide exercise programs; heat, cold, and whirlpool treatments to relieve pain; and hand splints and adaptive equipment to improve function and independence. O.T.'s have a bachelor's degree plus 6 months of specialized training. The costs of occupational therapy will be paid in part by Medicare if the patient is referred as an outpatient by a doctor or in full if the patient is in a hospital or skilled nursing facility.

189

Speech-language pathologists are concerned with speech and language problems while **audiologists** are interested in hearing disorders. Some specialists work in both areas. They test and evaluate patients, and they plan therapy to restore as much normal function as possible. Many speech-language pathologists work with stroke victims, those who have dementia, patients with diseases of the nervous system, and people who have had their vocal cords removed. Many audiologists work with older people whose hearing may be failing. They recommend hearing aids when needed and sometimes dispense them. Speech-language pathologists and audiologists have at least a master's degree. Most of them are licensed by the state in which they practice. Medicare generally will cover the services of speech-language pathologists and audiologists.

Social workers in health care settings alert patients to community services which might be useful, arrange for counseling when necessary, and help patients and their families handle problems related to physical and mental illness and disability. Older people might by referred to social workers by various health providers or their local governments. A social worker's education may range from a bachelor's degree to a doctorate. Most of them have a master's degree (M.S.W.). Medicare does not cover services provided by social workers unless they work in a hospital setting.

Dental Care

Dentists (D.D.S. or D.M.D.) treat oral conditions such as gum disease and tooth decay. They do regular checkups, give routine dental and preventive care, fill cavities, remove teeth, provide dentures, and check for cancers in the mouth. Dentists can prescribe medication and perform surgery. A

190

general dentist might refer patients to a specialist such as an oral surgeon, who does difficult tooth removals and surgery on the jaw; an endodontist, who is an expert on root canals; or a periodontist, who is especially knowledgeable about gum diseases. Medicare will not pay for any dental care except for surgery on the jaw or facial bones.

Dental hygienists (R.D.H.) examine, clean and polish teeth. They also take X-rays and teach patients about proper dental care. Although hygienists' duties vary according to state law, they almost always work under the supervision of a dentist. Most hygienists have at least 2 years of formal training and all are licensed by the state in which they practice. Medicare does not pay for their services.

Dental assistants help dentists and dental hygienists in the dental office. They may process X-rays, prepare the patient for examination, schedule appointments or assist the dentist while he or she works. Dental assistants may have some formal training or they may learn their responsibilities on the job. Their services are not covered by Medicare.

Eye Care

Ophthalmologists (M.D.) are M.D.'s or D.O.'s who specialize in the diagnosis and treatment of diseases of the eye. They also prescribe eyeglasses and contact lenses. Like other M.D.'s, ophthalmologists can prescribe drugs and perform surgery. They often treat older people who have glaucoma and cataracts. Medicare helps pay for all medically necessary surgery or treatment of eye diseases and for examinations and eyeglasses to correct vision after cataract surgery. But it will not pay for routine examinations, eyeglasses or contact lenses.

Optometrists (O.D.) generally have a bachelor's degree plus 4 years of graduate training at a school of optometry.

They are trained to diagnose eye abnormalities and prescribe, supply and adjust eyeglasses and contact lenses. In several states optometrists are authorized to use drugs to treat eye disease, and in most states they can use drugs to diagnose eye abnormalities. An optometrist may refer patients to an ophthalmologist or other medical specialist in cases requiring medication or surgery. Medicare pays for only a limited number of optometric services.

Opticians fit, supply and adjust eyeglasses and contact lenses which have been prescribed by an ophthalmologist or optometrist. They cannot examine or test the eyes, or prescribe glasses or drugs. Opticians are licensed in 22 states and may have formal training. Traditionally, however, most opticians learn their skills during on-the-job training.

Muscle, Bone, and Foot Care

Orthopedists (M.D. or D.O.) are surgeons who operate on and treat problems of the bones, joints, muscles, ligaments and tendons.

Podiatrists (D.P.M.) diagnose, treat and prevent diseases and injuries of the foot. They may do surgery, make devices to correct or prevent foot problems, provide toenail care, and prescribe certain drugs. A podiatrist is not licensed to treat diseases or injuries of any other part of the body. Podiatrists complete 4 years of professional school and, once they have been licensed, Medicare will cover the cost of their services except routine foot care. (However, routine foot care is covered if it is necessary because of diabetic complications).

Mental Health Care

Psychiatrists (M.D.) are M.D.'s or D.O.'s who treat people with mental and emotional difficulties. They can prescribe medication and counsel patients, as well as perform diagnostic tests to determine if there are physical problems. Medicare will pay for a portion of both inpatient and outpatient psychiatric costs.

Clinical psychologists (PH.D.) are called "doctor" because they have a doctoral degree in psychology. They are not medical doctors, but they counsel people with mental and emotional problems. (Some clinical psychologists who have a master's degree, but not a Ph.D., also work with patients, but they do not use the title "doctor".) The services of a clinical psychologist are not covered by Medicare except when they are performed in connection with the services of a psychiatrist or other M.D.

These are only a few of the health professionals who provide care to people of all ages. They are especially important to the elderly, some of whom require a great deal of medical attention. Ideally, all health professionals will work together to provide older people with care that is comprehensive, efficient, cost-effective and compassionate.

Selecting a Health Professional

Finding the health professional who best suits your needs may take time and effort. A good place to start is with friends and relatives who may recommend the health professional they use. Other possible sources of referrals are teaching hospitals, medical schools, dental schools, other health professionals, professional societies, or local consumer groups that may have done research to provide such information. For information about a specific health professional's education and specialties, you could call his or her office and ask or check your library for professional membership directories such as the *American Medical Association Directory* and the *Directory of Medical Specialists*. The Yellow Pages also lists health professionals by specialties.

When you have collected a list of candidates, call their offices to get information about what is particularly important to you. For example, you might ask:

- "How much will services cost and when are payments due?"
- "Is it possible to arrange a special payment schedule to fit my budget?"
- "Does the professional accept the type of insurance that I carry? Does he or she accept Medicare or Medicaid assignments? If so, for what services?"
- "Does the professional employ or recommend the use of other health professionals, such as physician's assistants or nurse practitioners?"
- "Is the office located near public transportation?"
- "What are the office hours?"
- "How does the office respond to emergencies after office hours?"
- "Is another professional on call when the doctor is unavailable?"

Deciphering Doctor Talk

Prefixes

a, an = without, not
ad = near
anti = against
endo(o) = within
ep(i) = on, upon, over
hyper = above, over, excessive
hypo = below, under, deficient
inter = between
intra = within
macro = large
micro = small
peri = around
pre = before, in front of
poly = many

Combining Forms

angio, angi = blood or lymph
     vessel
arterio = artery
arthro = joint
brady = slow
cardio = heart
chole, cholo = bile
colo = colon
cysto, cystido = sac, cyst, bladder
dys = difficult, painful
  abnormal
glyco = sugar
hema, hemo, hemato = blood
hepato = liver
hystero = uterus
leuco, leuko = white
lipo = fat
meno = menses
nephro = kidney
osteo = bone
pneumato, pneuma = air, gas
rhino = nose

sclero = hard
tachy = swift, rapid
veno = vein

Suffixes

algia = pain
cyte = cell
ectomy = excision of
emia = blood
itis = inflammation of
megaly = very large
oma = tumor, swelling
osis = disease, morbid process
ostomy = artificial opening
otomy, tomy = incision into
pathy = disease of
pnea = breathing
rhage, rhagia = bleeding,
     bursting forth
rhea = flow
uria = urine

By combining root words with prefixes and suffixes, words such as the following are formed:

arteriosclerosis = hardening of
    the arteries
bradycardia = slowness of the
    heartbeat
colostomy = surgical creation of
    an opening between
    the colon and the
    surface of the body
dyspnea = difficult or painful
    breathing
glycosuria = presence of sugar
    in the urine
hemorrhage = escape of blood
    from the vessels;
    bleeding

hepatitis = inflammation of the liver

hepatomegaly = enlargement of the liver

hyperlipemia = excessive fat in the blood

hysterectomy = removal of the uterus

intravenous = within a vein or veins

leucocyte = white blood cell

lipoma = a fatty tumor

macrocyst = a large cyst

neuralgia = severe sharp pain along the course of a nerve

periangioma = a tumor which surrounds a blood vessel

rhinitis = inflammation of the nasal passages

Common Abbreviations and Symbols
Used in Writing Prescriptions

Abbreviation	Meaning	Abbreviation	Meaning
A^2	both ears	OS	left eye
aa	of each	OU	each eye
ac	before meals	pc	after meals
AD	right ear	PM	evening
AL	left ear	po	by mouth
AM	morning	prn	as needed
AS	left ear	$\bar{q}$	every
bid	twice a day	qd	once a day
$\bar{c}$	with	qid	four times a day
cap	capsule	qod	every other day
cc or cm³	cubic centimeter	$\bar{s}$	without
disp	dispense	Sig	label as follows
dtd#	give this number	sl	under the tongue
ea	each	SOB	shortness of breath
ext	for external use		
gtts	drops	sol	solution
gutta	drop	ss	half-unit
h	hour	stat	at once, first dose
HS	bedtime	susp	suspension
M ft	make	tab	tablet
mitt#	give this number	tid	three times a day
ml	milliliter	top	apply topically
O	pint	ung or ungt	ointment
O_2	both eyes	UT	under the tongue
OD	right eye	ut dict	as directed
OJ	orange juice	x	times
OL	left eye		

Side Effects of Most Commonly Prescribed Prescription Drugs

Generic Name	Type of Drug	Side Effects
Acetaminophen w/Codeine	Analgesic	Constipation; dizziness; drowsiness; dry mouth; flushing; light headedness; nausea, rash; sweating; urine retention; vomiting; anxiety; bleeding or bruising; breathing difficulties; excitation; fatigue; jaundice; low blood sugar; palpitations; rapid or slow heartbeat; rash; restlessness; sore throat; tremors; weakness
Amitriptyline	Antidepressant	Agitation; blurred vision; confusion; constipation; cramps; diarrhea; dizziness; drowsiness; dry mouth; fatigue; headache; heartburn; increased sensitivity to light; insomnia; loss of appetite; nausea; peculiar tastes; restlessness; sweating; vomiting; weakness; weight gain or loss; bleeding; convulsions; difficult urination; enlarged or painful breasts (in both sexes); fainting; fever; fluid retention; hair loss; hallucinations; high or low blood pressure; imbalance; impotence; jaundice; mood changes; mouth sores; nervousness; nightmares; numbness in fingers or toes; palpitations; psychosis; ringing in the ears; seizures; skin rash; sleep disorders; sore throat; stroke; tremors; uncoordinated movements
Amoxicillin	Antibiotic	Diarrhea; nausea; vomiting; difficult breathing; fever; joint pain; mouth sores; rash; rectal and vaginal itching; severe diarrhea; sore throat; superinfection

Generic Name	Type of Drug	Side Effects
Ampicillin	Antibiotic	Diarrhea; nausea; vomiting; abdominal pain; black tongue; bruising, cough; difficult breathing; fever; mouth irritation; rash; rectal and vaginal itching; severe diarrhea; sore throat; superinfection
Aspirin w/Codeine	Analgesic	Confusion; constipation; dizziness; drowsiness; euphoria; flushing; headache; indigestion; itching; light-headedness; loss of appetite; nausea; slight blood loss; vomiting; black, tarry stools; breathing difficulties; jaundice; palpitations; rapid or slow heartbeat; ringing in the ears; skin rash; tremors; ulcers; urine retention
Chlordiazepoxide	Tranquilizer	Confusion; constipation; depression; dizziness; drooling; drowsiness; dry mouth; fainting; fatigue; fluid retention; headache; heartburn; insomnia; loss of appetite; menstrual irregularities; nausea; sweating; blood disorders; blurred vision; decrease or increase in sex drive; difficult breathing; difficult urination; double vision; excitation; fever; hallucinations; jaundice; low blood pressure; rash; slow heart rate; slurred speech; sore throat; stimulation; tremors; weakness
Chlorpromazine	Psychogenic	Blurred vision; constipation; decreased sweating; diarrhea; discoloration of the urine; dizziness; drooling; drowsiness; dry mouth; fainting; fatigue; jitteriness; low blood pressure; menstrual irregularities; nasal congestion; restlessness; sun sensitivity; tremors; vomiting; weight gain; blood disorders; breast enlargement; bruising; convulsions; darkened skin; difficulty with swallowing or breathing; fever; heart attack; im-

Generic Name	Type of Drug	Side Effects
Chlorpromazine (continued)		potence; involuntary movements of the face, mouth, jaw and tongue; jaundice; low or high blood sugar; palpitations; psychosis; rash; sleep disorders; sore throat; uncoordinated movements; visual disturbances
Chlorthalidone	Antihypertensive	Constipation; cramps; diarrhea; dizziness; drowsiness; headache; heartburn; loss of appetite; nausea; restlessness; sun sensitivity; vomiting; blood disorders; blurred vision; bruising; elevated blood sugar; elevated uric acid; fever; jaundice; mood changes; muscle spasm; rash; palpitations; sore throat; tingling in the fingers and toes; weakness; weak pulse
Diphenoxylate w/Atropine	Antidiarrheal	Blurred vision; constipation; dizziness; drowsiness; dry mouth; fever; flushing; headache; increased heart rate; itching; loss of appetite; nervousness; sedation; sweating; swollen gums; abdominal pain; bloating; breathing difficulties; coma; depression; difficult urination; euphoria; fever; hives; numbness in fingers or toes; palpitations; rash; severe nausea; vomiting; weakness
Dipyridamole	Vasodilator	Cramps; dizziness; fainting; fatigue; flushing; headache; nausea; weakness; rash; worsening of chest pain (mainly at start of therapy)
Erythromycin	Antibiotic	Abdominal cramps; black tongue; cough; diarrhea; fatigue; irritation of the mouth; loss of appetite; nausea; vomiting; fever; hearing loss; jaundice; rash; rectal and vaginal itching; superinfection

Generic Name	Type of Drug	Side Effects
Conjugated Estrogens	Estrogen	Bleeding; bloating; change in sexual desire; cramps; depression diarrhea; dizziness; headache; increased sensitivity to sunlight; loss of appetite; nausea; swelling of ankles and feet; vomiting
Furosemide	Cardiovascular	Blurred vision; constipation; cramping; diarrhea; dizziness; headache; itching; loss of appetite; muscle spasm; nausea; sore mouth; stomach upset; sun sensitivity; vomiting; weakness; anemia; blood disorders; bruising; dry mouth; gout; jaundice; loss of appetite; low blood pressure; muscle cramps; palpitations; pancreatitis; rash; ringing in the ears; rise in blood sugar; sore throat; thirst; tingling in the fingers and toes
Hydralazine	Hypertensive	Constipation; diarrhea; difficult urination; dizziness; flushing; headache; loss of appetite; muscle cramps; nasal congestion; nausea; vomiting; anemia; anxiety; blood disorders; bruising; chest pain; confusion; cramping; depression; fever; fluid retention; itching; liver damage; numbness or tingling in fingers or toes; palpitations; rapid heart rate; rash; shortness of breath; sore throat; tenderness in joints
Hydrochlorothiazide	Diuretic	Constipation; cramps; diarrhea; dizziness; drowsiness; headache; heartburn; itching; loss of appetite; nausea; restlessness; sun sensitivity; vomiting; blood disorders; blurred vision; bruising; elevated blood sugar; elevated uric acid; fever; jaundice; muscle spasm; palpitations; skin rash; sore throat; tingling in fingers and toes; weakness

Generic Name	Type of Drug	Side Effects
Imipramine	Antidepressant	Agitation; anxiety; black tongue; blurred vision; confusion; constipation; cramps; diarrhea; dizziness; drowsiness; dry mouth; fatigue; flushing; headache; heartburn; increased sensitivity to light; insomnia; loss of appetite; nausea; peculiar tastes; restlessness; stomach upset; sweating; urine color change; vomiting; weakness; bleeding; convulsions; difficult urination; enlarged or painful breasts (in both sexes); fainting; fever; fluid retention; hair loss; hallucinations; heart attack; high or low blood pressure; imbalance; impotence; jaundice; mood changes; mouth sores; nervousness; psychosis; nightmares; numbness in fingers or toes; palpitations; rash; ringing in the ears; sleep disorders; sore throat; stroke; testicular swelling; tremors; uncoordinated movements; weight loss or gain
Isosorbide Dinitrate	Cardiovascular	Dizziness; flushing; headache; nausea; vomiting; fainting spells; low blood pressure; palpitations; rash; restlessness; sweating; weakness
Meprobamate	Tranquilizer	Blurred vision; diarrhea; dizziness; dry mouth; headache; nausea; sedation; vomiting; weakness; bruising; clumsiness; confusion; convulsions; difficult breathing; euphoria; fainting; fever; fluid retention; kidney damage; low blood pressure; nightmares; numbness or tingling; palpitations; rash; slurred speech; sore throat; stimulation; weakness

PREVENTIVE HEALTH SERVICES

Family Planning

- *Planned Parenthood Federation of America, Inc.*
  810 Seventh Avenue
  New York, New York 10019
  (212) 541-7800

- *National Family Planning and Reproductive Health Association, Inc.*
  Suite 350
  425 Thirteenth Street, N.W.
  Washington, D.C. 20004
  (202) 783-1560

- *American College of Obstetricians and Gynecologists*
  Resource Center
  Suite 2700
  1 East Wacker Drive
  Chicago, Illinois 60601
  (312) 222-1600

- *National Clearinghouse for Family Planning Information*
  6110 Executive Blvd., Suite 250
  Rockville, Maryland 29852
  (301) 881-9400

Pregnancy and Infant Care

- *Office of Maternal and Child Health*
  Program Services Branch
  Bureau of Community Health Services
  Health Services Administration
  Room 7A20, Parklawn
  5600 Fishers Lane
  Rockville, Maryland 20857
  (301) 443-4273

- *National Foundation--March of Dimes*
  Public Health Education Department
  1275 Mamaroneck Avenue
  White Plains, New York 10605
  (914) 428-7100

- *American College of Obstetricians and Gynecologists*
  Resource Center
  Suite 2700
  1 East Wacker Drive
  Chicago, Illinois 60601
  (312) 222-1600

- *American Academy of Pediatrics*
  1801 Hinman Avenue
  Evanston, Illinois 60204
  (312) 869-4255

Immunizations

- *Center for Disease Control*
  Bureau of State Services
  Technical Information Services
  Center for Disease Control
  Atlanta, Georgia 30333
  (404) 452-4021

- *National Institute of Child Health and Human*
  Development
  Office of Research Reporting
  Room 2A34, Building 31
  National Institutes of Health
  Bethesda, Maryland 20205
  (301) 496-5133

Sexually Transmissible Diseases

- *Center for Disease Control*
  Bureau of State Services
  Technical Information Services
  Center for Disease Control
  Atlanta, Georgia 30333
  (404) 452-4021

- *American Social Health Association*
  260 Sheridan Avenue
  Palo Alto, California 94306
  (415) 321-5134

- *VD National Hotline*
  260 Sheridan Avenue
  Palo Alto, California 94306
  (800) 227-8922

High Blood Pressure and Heart Disease

- *National High Blood Pressure Information Center*
  Suite 1300
  7910 Woodmont Avenue
  Bethesda, Maryland 20014
  (301) 652-7700

- *National Heart, Lung, and Blood Institute*
  Public Inquiries Office
  Room 4A21, Building 31
  National Institutes of Health
  Bethesda, Maryland 20205
  (301) 496-4236

- *American Heart Association*
  7320 Greenville Avenue
  Dallas, Texas 75231
  (214) 750-5300
  (or local chapters)

- *Consumer Information Center*
  Pueblo, Colorado 81009
  (303) 544-5277, ext. 370

HEALTH PROTECTION

Toxic Agent Control

- *Center for Disease Control*
  Chronic Diseases Division
  Bureau of Epidemiology
  Building 1, Room 5127
  Center for Disease Control
  Atlanta, Georgia 30333
  (404) 329-3165

- *Environmental Protection Agency*
  Office of Public Awareness
  Environmental Protection Agency
  401 M Street, S.W.
  Mail Code: A-107
  Washington, D.C. 20460
  (202) 755-0700

- *National Institute of Environmental Health Sciences*
  National Institutes of Health
  Post Office Box 12233
  Research Triangle Park, North Carolina 27709
  (919) 541-3345

- *American Lung Association*
  1740 Broadway
  New York, New York 10019
  (212) 245-8000
  (or local chapter)

Occupational Safety and Health

- *Occupational Safety and Health Administration*
  Office of Public and Consumer Affairs
  U.S. Department of Labor (Room N3637)
  200 Constitution Avenue, N.W.
  Washington, D.C. 20210
  (202) 523-8151

- *Clearinghouse for Occupational Safety and Health*
  National Institute for Occupational Safety and Health
  Center for Disease Control
  Robert A. Taft Laboratory
  4676 Columbia Parkway
  Cincinnati, Ohio 45226
  (513) 684-8326

- *National Safety Council*
  444 North Michigan Avenue
  Chicago, Illinois 60611
  (312) 527-4800

- *American Industrial Hygiene Association*
  475 Wolf Ledges Parkway
  Akron, Ohio 44311
  (216) 762-7294

- *American Occupational Medical Association*
  Suite 2240
  150 North Wacker Drive
  Chicago, Illinois 60606
  (312) 782-2166

Accidental Injury Control

- *Consumer Product Safety Commission*
  Consumer Education and Awareness Division
  5401 Westbard Avenue

207

Washington, D.C. 20207
(202) 492-6576
(or local Poison Control Centers)

- *Department of Transportation*
  General Services Division (NAD-42)
  National Highway Traffic Safety Administration
  Department of Transportation
  400 Seventh Street, S.W. (Room 4423)
  Washington, D.C. 20590
  (202) 426-0874
  ATTN: E. Kitts

- *National Safety Council*
  444 North Michigan Avenue
  Chicago, Illinois 60611
  (312) 527-4800

- *American Red Cross*
  National Headquarters
  18th and E Streets, N.W.
  Washington, D.C. 20006
  (202) 857-3555

Community Water Supply Fluoridation

- *Center for Disease Control*
  Dental Disease Prevention Activity (E107)
  Center for Disease Control
  Atlanta, Georgia 30333
  (404) 262-6631

- *National Institute of Dental Research*
  Public Inquiries Office
  Room 2C34, Building 31
  National Institutes of Health
  Bethesda, Maryland 20205
  (301) 496-4261

- *American Dental Association*
  Bureau of Health, Education and Audiovisual
  Services
  American Dental Association
  211 East Chicago Avenue
  Chicago, Illinois 60611
  (312) 440-2593

Infectious Agent Control

- *Center for Disease Control*
  Public Inquiries
  Management Analysis and Service Office
  Building 4, Room B2
  Center for Disease Control
  Atlanta, Georgia 30333
  (404) 329-3534

- *National Institute of Allergy and Infectious Diseases*
  Office of Research Reporting and Public Response
  Room 7A32, Building 31
  National Institutes of Health
  Bethesda, Maryland 20205
  (301) 496-5717

HEALTH PROMOTION

Smoking Cessation

- *Technical Information Center for Smoking and Health*
  Office on Smoking and Health
  Department of Health, Education and Welfare
  Room 1-16, Park Building
  5600 Fishers Lane

Rockville, Maryland 20857
(301) 443-1690

- *Office of Cancer Communications*
  National Cancer Institute
  Room 10A18, Building 31
  National Institutes of Health
  Bethesda, Maryland 20205
  (301) 496-5583

- *American Cancer Society*
  Public Information Department
  777 Third Avenue
  New York, New York 10017
  (212) 371-2900, ext. 254
  (or local chapter)

- *American Lung Association*
  1740 Broadway
  New York, New York 10019
  (212) 245-8000
  (or local chapter)

- *American Heart Association*
  7320 Greenville Avenue
  Dallas, Texas 75231
  (214) 750-5300
  (or local chapter)

Reducing Misuse of Alcohol and Drugs

- *National Clearinghouse on Alcohol Information*
  Post Office Box 2345
  Rockville, Maryland 20852
  (301) 468-2600

- *National Clearinghouse on Drug Abuse Information*
  Room 10A53, Parklawn Building
  5600 Fishers Lane

Rockville, Maryland 20857
(301) 443-6500

- *National Council on Alcoholism*
  733 Third Avenue
  New York, New York 10017
  (212) 986-4433

- *Alcoholics Anonymous*
  General Services Office (6th Floor)
  468 Park Avenue South
  New York, New York 10016
  (212) 686-1100
  ATTN: Public Information Department

Improved Nutrition

- *Food and Drug Administration*
  Office of Consumer Communications (HFG-10)
  Food and Drug Administration
  Room 15B32, Parklawn Building
  5600 Fishers Lane
  Rockville, Maryland 20857
  (301) 443-3170

- *U.S. Department of Agriculture*
  Human Nutrition Center SEA
  Room 421A
  U.S. Department of Agriculture
  Washington, D.C. 20250
  (202) 447-7854

- *Consumer Information Center*
  Pueblo, Colorado 81009
  (303) 544-5277, ext. 370

- *Nutrition Foundation*
  Suite 300
  888 Seventeenth Street, N.W.
  Washington, D.C. 20006
  (202) 872-0778

- *National Nutrition Education Clearinghouse*
  Suite 1110
  2140 Shattuck Avenue
  Berkeley, California 94704
  (415) 548-1363

Exercise and Fitness

- *President's Council on Physical Fitness and Sports*
  Department of Health, Education and Welfare
  Room 3030, Donohoe Building
  400 Sixth Street, S.W.
  Washington, D.C. 20201
  (202) 755-7947

- *American Alliance for Health, Physical Education, Recreation and Dance*
  Promotions Unit
  1201 Sixteenth Street, N.W.
  Washington, D.C. 20036
  (202) 833-5534

- *American College of Sports Medicine*
  1440 Monroe Street
  Madison, Wisconsin 53706
  (608) 262-3632

Stress Control

- *National Clearinghouse for Mental Health Information*
  National Institute of Mental Health
  Room 11A33, Parklawn Building
  5600 Fishers Lane
  Rockville, Maryland 20857
  (301) 443-4517

- *Mental Health Association*
  1800 North Kent Street
  Arlington, Virginia 22209
  (703) 528-6405
  (or local chapters)

- *Public Affairs Committee, Inc.*
  Room 1101
  381 Park Avenue South
  New York, New York 10016
  (212) 683-4331

- *Blue Cross and Blue Shield Associations*
  Public Relations Office
  840 North Lake Shore Drive
  Chicago, Illinois 60611
  (312) 440-5955

GENERAL INFORMATION SOURCES

Public Health Service

- *Bureau of Health Education*
  Building 14
  Center for Disease Control
  Atlanta, Georgia 30333
  (404) 329-3111

- *Office of Health Information and Health Promotion*
  Office of the Surgeon General
  Department of Health, Education and Welfare
  (Room 721BHHH)
  200 Independence Avenue, S.W.
  Washington, D.C.
  (202) 472-5370

National Organizations

- *National Association of Community Health Centers, Inc.*
  Suite 420
  1625 Eye Street, N.W.
  Washington, D.C. 20006
  (202) 833-9280

- *National Center for Health Education*
  211 Sutter Street (4th Floor)
  San Francisco, California 94108
  (415) 781-6144

State and Local Levels

- *Contact your family physician*
- *Contact your local health department*
- *Contact your county's cooperative extension service*

Suggested Body Weights

Range of Acceptable Weights

Height (feet-inches)	Men (Pounds)	Women (Pounds)
4'10"		92-119
4'11"		94-122
5'0"		96-125
5'1"		99-128
5'2"	112-141	102-131
5'3"	115-144	105-134
5'4"	118-148	108-138
5'5"	121-152	111-142
5'6"	124-156	114-146
5'7"	128-161	118-150
5'8"	132-166	122-154
5'9"	136-170	126-158
5'10"	140-174	130-163
5'11"	144-179	134-168
6'0"	148-184	138-173
6'1"	152-189	
6'2"	156-194	
6'3"	160-199	
6'4"	164-204	

NOTE: Height without shoes; weight without clothes.

Exercise Pulse Rates

Age	Target Zone
20	120-150
25	117-146
30	114-142
35	111-138
40	108-135
45	105-131
50	102-127
55	99-123
60	96-120
65	93-116
70	90-113

"Target zone" is the pulse or heart rate in beats per minute. Exercise that sustains that target zone level for 30 minutes should be undertaken at least three times a week. Persons over 40 who have not been exercising regularly should consult a doctor before embarking on such a program.

Source: Exercise and Your Heart; National Heart, Lung and Blood Institute.

Blood Pressure Classifications

Diastolic Blood Pressure
(the lower of the two numbers)

Reading	Category
Less than 85	Normal blood pressure
85 to 89	High normal blood pressure
90 to 104	Mild hypertension
105 to 114	Moderate hypertension
115 or more	Severe hypertension

Systolic Pressure
(the higher of the two numbers)

Reading	Category
Less than 140	Normal blood pressure
140 to 159	Borderline isolated systolic hypertension
160 or more	Isolated systolic hypertension

These categories are for persons 18 and older.

Source: The 1984 "Report of the Joint National Committee on Detection, Evaluation and Treatment of High Blood Pressure."

Calorie and Fat Guide To
Some Fast Foods

Item	Total Calories	Calories In Fat
Burger King		
Cheeseburger	305	117
French fries, large	428	180
French fries, regular	214	90
Hamburger	252	81
Hamburger, Whopper	606	288
Hot dog	291	153
Shake, vanilla	331	86
Whaler	486	414
Kentucky Fried Chicken		
Original Recipe, dinner	830	414
Individual pieces (original recipe)		
drumstick	136	72
thigh	276	171
wing	151	90
9 pieces	1892	1044
Coleslaw	110	53
Potato, mashed w/gravy	74	18
McDonald's		
Big Mac	541	283
Cheeseburger	306	120
Egg McMuffin	352	180
Eggs, scrambled	161	107
Filet O'Fish	402	204
French fries	211	95
Hamburger	257	85
Hot cakes w/butter and syrup	472	81
McDonaldland Cookies (1 box)	292	95
Pie, apple	295	165
Pie, cherry	296	158

Item	Total Calories	Calories In Fat
Quarter Pounder	418	185
Quarter Pounder w/cheese	518	257
Sausage, pork	191	155
Shake, chocolate	324	76
Shake, strawberry	346	77
Shake, vanilla	324	70

Pizza Hut
(Figures are for 3 slices;
½ of a 10-inch pizza)
Thin 'n' Crispy

Beef	490	171
Cheese	450	135
Pepperoni	430	153
Pork	520	207
Supreme		

Thick 'n' Chewy

Beef	620	180
Cheese	560	126
Pepperoni	560	162
Pork	640	207
Supreme	640	198

Taco Bell

Bean burrito	343	108
Beef burrito	466	189
Beefy tostada	291	135
Bellbeefer	221	63
Bellbeefer w/cheese	278	108
Burrito Supreme	457	198
Combination burrito	404	144
Enchirito	454	189
Pintos 'n' Cheese	168	45
Taco	186	72
Tostada	179	54

Other Mexican Foods
Enchilada

beef	260	110

Item	Total Calories	Calories In Fat
beef topped w/cheese	340	170
cheese	280	130
Guacamole (½ cup)	140	130
Refried beans (½ cup)	150	45
Taco salad	234	130
Tamale	115	45
Tortilla	40	10
Wendy's		
Cheeseburger		
single	520	270
triple	940	531
Chili con carne	250	63
French fries	340	153
Hamburger		
single	440	225
double	630	306
triple	780	405
Shake, chocolate	390	135

Calorie Content Of
Everyday Foods

Fruit Drinks   **Calories**

Apple juice, canned, ½ cup 60
Cranberry juice cocktail, ½ cup 80
Grape drink, ½ cup 70
Lemonade, frozen concentrate, sweetened,
   ready-to-serve, ½ cup 55
Orange juice, fresh, ½ cup 55
   canned, unsweetened, ½ cup 60
   frozen concentrate, ready-to-serve, ½ cup 55
Pineapple, canned, unsweetened, ½ cup 70
Peach nectar, ½ cup 60
Pear nectar, ½ cup 65

Carbonated Beverages   **Calories**

Cola-type, 8-ounce glass 95
   12-ounce can or bottle 145
Fruit flavors, 10-13% sugar, 8 ounce glass 115
   12-ounce can or bottle 170
Ginger ale, 8-ounce glass 75
   12-ounce can or bottle 115

Alcoholic Beverages   **Calories**

Beer, 3.6% alcohol, 8-ounce glass 100
   12-ounce can or bottle 150
   Whiskey, gin, rum, vodka
   80-proof, 1½-ounce jigger 95
   90-proof, 1½-ounce jigger 110
Wines, table (Chablis, claret, Rhine wine, sauterne, etc.),
   3½-ounce glass 85

Bread   **Calories**

Cracked wheat, 18 slices per pound loaf, 1 slice 65
Raisin, 18 slices per pound loaf, 1 slice 65
Rye, 18 slices per pound loaf, 1 slice 60
White
   soft crumb, 18 slices per pound loaf, 1 slice 70
   firm crumb, 20 slices per pound loaf, 1 slice 65
Whole wheat
   soft crumb, 16 slices per pound loaf, 1 slice 65
   firm crumb, 18 slices per pound loaf, 1 slice 60

Cereals   **Calories**

Bran flakes, (40% bran) 1 ounce 85
   with raisins, 1 ounce 80
Corn, puffed, presweetened, 1 ounce (about 1 cup) 115

Corn flakes, plain, 1 ounce (about 1 1/6 cups) 110
    sugar coated, 1 ounce (about 2/3 cup).......................110
Farina, cooked, quick-cooking, ¾ cup 80
Oats, puffed, plain, 1 ounce (about 1 1/6 cups) 115
    sugar-coated, 1 ounce (about 4/5 cup).....................115
Oatmeal or rolled oats, cooked, ¾ cup 100
Rice, flakes, 1 ounce (about 1 cup)...........................110
    puffed, 1 ounce (about 2 cups)............................115
Wheat, puffed, 1 ounce (about 1⅞ cups) 105
    rolled, cooked, ¾ cup.....................................135
    shredded, plain, 1 ounce, (1 large buscuit or ½ cup bite size) ...100
    flakes, 1 ounce (about 1 cup) 100

Candies   Calories

Caramels, (1 ounce) 3 medium 115
Chocolate creams, 35 to a pound, 2 to 3 pieces (1 ounce) 125
Chocolate, milk, sweetened, 1-ounce bar 145
Chocolate mints, 20 to a pound, 1 to 2 mints (1 ounce)..........115
Fudge, vanilla or chocolate
    plain, 1 ounce..115
    with nuts, 1 ounce 120
Gumdrops, about 2½ large or 20 small (1 ounce) 100
Hard candy, three or four ¾-inch-diameter candy balls (1 ounce)..110
Jellybeans, 10 (1 ounce) 105
Marshmallows, 4 large 90

Other Sweets   Calories

Chocolate, bittersweet, 1-ounce square 135
    semisweet, 1-ounce square 145
Chocolate sirup, thin type, 1 tablespoon 45
    fudge type, 1 tablespoon 60
Cranberry sauce, canned, 1 tablespoon.........................25
Honey, 1 tablespoon 65
Jam, preserves, 1 tablespoon..................................55
Jelly, marmalade, 1 tablespoon................................50
Molasses, 1 tablespoon 50
Sirup, table blends, 1 tablespoon 55
Sugar, white, granulated, or brown (packed) 1 teaspoon 15

Pies   Calories

Apple, ⅛ of 9-inch pie 300
Blueberry, ⅛ of 9-inch pie...................................285
Cherry, ⅛ of 9-inch pie 310
Chocolate meringue, ⅛ of 9-inch pie 285
Custard, plain, ⅛ of 9-inch pie 250
Lemon meringue, ⅛ of 9-inch pie 270
Mince, ⅛ of 9-inch pie.......................................320
Peach, ⅛ of 9-inch pie.......................................300
Pecan, ⅛ of 9-inch pie 430

Other Desserts
Calories

Apple betty, ½ cup 160
Bread pudding, with raisins, ½ cup 250
Brownie, with nuts, 1¾-inches square, ⅞-inch thick 90
Custard, baked, ½ cup 150
Gelatin, plain, ½ cup 70
   with fruit, ½ cup 80
Ice cream, plain
   regular (about 10% fat), ½ cup 130
   rich (about 16% fat), ½ cup 165
Ice milk, hardened, ½ cup 100
   soft serve, ½ cup 135
Puddings
   cornstarch, vanilla, ½ cup 140
   chocolate, from a mix, ½ cup 160
   tapioca cream, ½ cup 110
Sherbet, ½ cup 130

Fats And Oils
Calories

Butter or margarine, 1 pat, 1-inch square, 1/3-inch thick 35
   1 tablespoon 100
Cooking fats, vegetable, 1 tablespoon 100
   lard, 1 tablespoon 115

Cream
Calories

Half & half (milk and cream), 1 tablespoon 20
   1 cup 315
Light, coffee or table, 1 tablespoon 30
Sour, 1 tablespoon 25
Whipped topping, pressurized, 1 tablespoon 10
Whipping, heavy, 1 tablespoon 50
   light, 1 tablespoon 45

Beef
Calories

Beef and vegetable stew, canned, 1 cup 195
   homemade, with lean beef, 1 cup 220
Beef potpie, home prepared, baked, ¼ of 9-inch pie 385
Chili con carne, canned, with beans, ½ cup 170
   without beans, ½ cup 240
Corned beef, canned, 3 ounces 185
Corned beef hash, 2/5 cup (3 ounces) 155
Dried beef, chipped, 1/3 cup (2 ounces) 115
   creamed, ½ cup 190
Hamburger, broiled, panbroiled, or sauteed
   regular, 3 ounces 245
   lean, 3 ounces 185
Oven roast, cooked, without bone
   cuts relatively fat, such as rib, lean and fat, 3 ounces 375

lean only, 3 ounces 205
cuts relatively lean, such as round, lean and fat, 3 ounces 220
lean only, 3 ounces 160
Pot roast, cooked, braised or simmered, without bone
lean and fat, 3 ounces 245
lean only, 3 ounces 165
Steak, broiled, without bone
cuts relatively fat, such as sirloin, lean and fat, 3 ounces 330
lean only, 3 ounces 175
cuts relatively lean, such as round, lean and fat, 3 ounces 220
lean only, 3 ounces 160
Veal cutlet, broiled, with bone, trimmed, 3 ounces 185
Veal roast, cooked, without bone, 3 ounces 230

Lamb   Calories

Loin chop, broiled, without bone
lean and fat, 3 ounces 305
lean only, 3 ounces 160
Leg, roasted, without bone
lean and fat, 3 ounces 235
lean only, 3 ounces 160
Shoulder, roasted, without bone
lean and fat, 3 ounces 285
lean only, 3 ounces 175

Pork   Calories

Bacon, broiled or fried, crisp, 2 thin slices 60
2 medium slices 85
Bacon, Canadian, cooked, one 3 3/8 x 3/16-inch slice 60
Chop, broiled without bone, lean and fat, 3 ounces 335
lean only, 3 ounces 230
Ham, cured, cooked, without bone, lean and fat, 3 ounces 245
lean only, 3 ounces 160
Roast, loin, cooked, without bone, lean and fat, 3 ounces 310
lean only, 3 ounces 215

Poultry   Calories

Chicken, roasted (no skin) breast, one-half 140
fried (no skin), breast, ½ 160
thigh, one 115
drumstick, one 80
canned, meat with broth, ½ cup (3½ ounces)................. 165
Poultry pie, home prepared, baked, ¼ of 9-inch pie.............. 410
Turkey, roasted (no skin) light meat, 3 ounces 135
dark meat, 3 ounces 160

Fish And Shellfish   Calories

Clams, shelled, canned, 3 medium clams and juice (3 ounces) 45
raw, meat only, 4 medium (3 ounces)........................ 65

Fish sticks, breaded, cooked, frozen,
  three 4 x 1 x ½-inch sticks (3 ounces) 150
Haddock, breaded, fried, 3 ounces (4 x 2½ x ½-inch fillet) 140
Ocean perch, breaded, fried, 3 ounces (4 x 2½ x ½-inch piece) . . . 195
Oysters, raw, meat only, ½ cup (6 to 10 medium) 80
Salmon, broiled or baked, 3 ounces 155
  canned, pink, 3/5 cup with liquid (3 ounces) 120
Sardines, canned in oil, drained, 7 medium (3 ounces) 170
Shrimp, canned, 27 medium (3 ounces) 100
Tunafish, canned in oil, drained, ½ cup (3 ounces) 170

Eggs
Calories

Fried in fat, large, one 95
Hard or soft cooked, "boiled", large, one 80
Omelet, plain, 1 large egg, milk, and fat for cooking 110
Poached, large, one 80
Scrambled in fat, 1 large egg and milk 110

Dried Beans And Peas
Calories

Baked beans, canned, with pork and tomatoe sauce, ½ cup 155
  with pork and sweet sauce, ½ cup 190
Limas, cooked, ½ cup 130
Red kidney beans, canned or cooked, ½ cup, with liquid 110

Milk
Calories

Buttermilk, 1 cup 100
Condensed, sweetened, undiluted, ½ cup 490
Evaporated, whole, undiluted, ½ cup 170
Lowfat, 2% fat, nonfat, milksolids added, 1 cup 125
Skim, 1 cup 85
Whole, 1 cup 150

Yogurt
Calories

Made from skim milk, 1 cup 125
Made from whole mile, 1 cup 140

Milk Beverages
Calories

Chocolate milkshake, one 12-ounce container 405
Cocoa, homemade, 1 cup 220
Malted milk, 1 cup 235

Soups
Calories

Canned, condensed, prepared with equal volume of water unless otherwise stated
Bean with bacon, 1 cup 175
Beef noodle, 1 cup 85
Bouillon, broth or consomme, 1 cup 15
Chicken noodle, 1 cup 75
Clam chowder, manhattan, 1 cup 80
Cream of chicken, with water, 1 cup 115

Minestrone, 1 cup 85
Pea, split, 1 cup 190
Tomato, with water, 1 cup 85
   with milk, 1 cup 160

Vegetables (Raw)   Calories

Cabbage, plain, shredded, chopped or sliced, ½ cup 10
Carrots, 7½ x 1⅛-inch carrot 30
   ½ cup, grated 25
Celery, three 5-inch stalks 10
Cucumbers, pared, 6 center slices, ⅛-inch thick 5
Lettuce, leaves, large, two 5
Tomatoes, 2 2/5-inch diameter tomato 20

Vegetables (cooked, canned or frozen)   Calories

Asparagus spears, 6 medium or ½ cup cut 20
Beans, green lima, ½ cup 90
   snap, green, wax or yellow, ½ cup 15
Beets, diced, sliced or small whole, ½ cup 30
Broccoli, chopped, ½ cup 25
Cabbage, ½ cup 15
Carrots, ½ cup 25
Cauliflower, flower buds, ½ cup 15
Corn, on cob, one 5-inch ear 70
   kernels, drained, ½ cup 70
   cream-style, ½ cup 105
Peas, green, ½ cup 65
Potatoes, baked, 2 1/3-inch diameter, 4¾-inch long, one 145
   boiled, 2½-inch diameter whole, one 90
   french fries, fresh, ten 1½ x ¼-inch pieces 215
   mashed, milk added, ½ cup 70
Sweetpotatoes, baked in skin, 5 x 2-inch, one 160
Tomatoes, ½ cup 30

Fruits (Raw)   Calories

Apples, 2¾-inch-diameter, one 80
Apricots, 3 (about ¼ pound) 55
Bananas, one 6 to 7-inch banana (about 1/3 pound) 85
Cantaloup, 5-inch melon, one-half 80
Grapefruit, white, half of a 3¾-inch fruit 45
Grapes, slip skin (concord, delaware, niagara, etc.) ½ cup ... 35
Honeydew melon, 2 x 7-inch wedge 50
Oranges, 2 5/8-inch orange 65
Peaches, slices, ½ cup 30
   whole, 2½-inch peach (about ¼ pound) 40
Pears, 3½ x 2½ inch, one 100
Pineapple, diced, ½ cup 40
Plums, damson, 1 inch (2 ounces), five 35
Raisins, packed, ½ cup 240
Tangerines, 2 3/8-inch tangerine (about ¼ pound), one 40